CARROTS 'N' CAKE

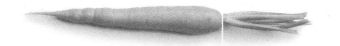

CARROTS 'N' CAKE

HEALTHY LIVING ONE CARROT AND CUPCAKE AT A TIME

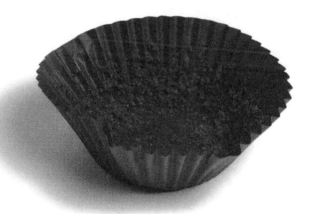

TINA HAUPERT

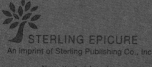

STERLING EPICURE
An Imprint of Sterling Publishing Co., Inc.

New York / London
www.sterlingpublishing.com

STERLING and the distinctive Sterling logo are registered trademarks of Sterling Publishing Co., Inc.

Library of Congress Cataloging-in-Publication Data

Haupert, Tina.
  Carrots 'N' cake : healthy living one carrot and cupcake at a time / Tina Haupert.
    p. cm.
  Includes index.
  ISBN 978-1-4027-7824-7 (pb-with flaps : alk. paper) 1. Nutrition. 2. Diet. 3. Physical fitness. 4. Cookbooks. I. Title.
  TX355.H417 2011
  613.2--dc22

                                        2010039033

10 9 8 7 6 5 4 3 2 1

Published by Sterling Publishing Co., Inc.
387 Park Avenue South, New York, NY 10016
© 2011 by Tina Haupert
Distributed in Canada by Sterling Publishing
c/o Canadian Manda Group, 165 Dufferin Street
Toronto, Ontario, Canada M6K 3H6
Distributed in the United Kingdom by GMC Distribution Services
Castle Place, 166 High Street, Lewes, East Sussex, England BN7 1XU
Distributed in Australia by Capricorn Link (Australia) Pty. Ltd.
P.O. Box 704, Windsor, NSW 2756, Australia

Sterling ISBN 978-1-4027-7824-7

For information about custom editions, special sales, premium and corporate purchases, please contact Sterling Special Sales Department at 800-805-5489 or specialsales@sterlingpublishing.com.

Designed by Barbara Balch

TO MY MOM

It's all about the cake.

CONTENTS

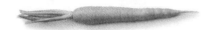

Every person is different. Your body mass, your metabolism, your endurance, etc. And everyone's eating habits are different as well. This book is a very personal book, and as such, the exercise routines and recipes worked for me, in finding a happy goal weight and exercise lifestyle. You should not take on any exercise recommendations without at least discussing it with your doctor first. The recipes and workout routines in this book reflect my personal lifestyle, and I came to them by way of local, trained personal trainers, and by trial and error by way of food. The conditioning exercises and the recipes have not been vetted by a registered dietitian or a medical doctor.

INTRODUCTION

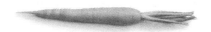

I t all started as a countdown to my wedding. I wasn't necessarily overweight, but I wanted to tone up and be in great shape by the time the big day arrived—nineteen months down the road. I had been using an online calorie and exercise tracker to keep myself accountable, and reading food blogs helped me to develop my own program.

When people ask me why I started blogging, I think they expect me to tell them that I wanted to save the world or inspire people to live a healthy lifestyle. I sometimes think they're a little disappointed when I explain that I started blogging for personal reasons and I really had no intention of people ever reading what I wrote.

Carrots 'N' Cake is a journal of my daily eats and workouts. For me, it is a creative extension of the online calorie and exercise tracker that I had been using prior to starting the blog.

I had been reading food blogs for a few months before I finally decided to take the leap to my own postings. *Self* magazine's *Eat Like Me* was the very first blog of its kind that I regularly read. A registered dietitian living in Boston documented her meals every day as an example of a healthy and balanced way to eat. The comments on her posts soon led me to the blog that I credit as the influence and motivation to start my own: *Kath Eats Real Food*. Kath documented her daily meals as she lost weight, but her blog posts were much more detailed than just a list of what she ate. She divulged her personal and home life, shared delicious recipes, reviewed products, and talked about the importance of incorporating fitness into her life. She really pulled me in. Soon, I was reading her blog three times a day! My mini-obsession with Kath's life eventually inspired me to start my own blog.

Kath leads a very healthy lifestyle. All of her meals are full of fresh produce, high-quality grains, and low-fat protein. She knows how to create a well-balanced meal and present it in such a way that inspired me to eat well myself. I wanted to eat as healthfully as Kath, but I knew that I couldn't give up some of my favorite foods, like cookies, cake, nachos, and wine. I'd be miserable if I couldn't have them. So, when I was thinking about what to call my blog and what angle I would write it from, I couldn't help but think about how to incorporate dessert into a balanced diet. I knew it could be done! It was all about balancing the "good" foods (carrots) with the "bad" foods (cake).

I thought having a blog that was devoted to achieving this balance of all kinds of food would distinguish my blog from Kath's. I loved her blog, but I knew that I had something different to offer. Basically, I thought, *If this woman can lose thirty pounds by recording her efforts on a blog, I bet I will have success doing the same thing.* I had nothing to lose by signing up for a free blog and giving it a try. Plus, at the time, I was looking for a hobby, so blogging fit right into my ample downtime.

I know—a hobby. You'd think I had enough to do, what with working full-time and planning a wedding, right? The truth is, I like to keep busy and I'm a good planner, so I took care of most of the tough stuff for the wedding in the early months of my engagement. I was never a stressed-out bridezilla. Mal, my fiance, had an active fantasy football team and liked to spend his downtime playing video games. I had lots of interests—I liked running, baking, and photography—but I'm easily bored, so I was looking for something to fill the extra hours. Blogging looked like a great hobby.

Typically, coming up with a name for a blog is somewhat difficult. I've heard of potential bloggers wracking their brains for weeks trying to think of a catchy, witty blog name that people will remember—and then it just comes to them while they're commuting to work or in the shower. *Carrots 'N' Cake* came to me while sitting in bed—just seconds after I decided that I'd start a blog. The name sort of signified that I was meant to blog. It was just so easy. *Carrots 'N' Cake* was just meant to be!

Even so, when I started to blog, I was sort of embarrassed about it. I didn't even tell Mal what I was doing for a few weeks! *Is this too weird?* I thought, *Taking photos of everything I eat and then writing about it?* Would people think I was strangely obsessed with food? I didn't think so—at least I hoped not. And once I got started, I found blogging to be fun and really motivating: I liked to see my progress on my blog, and, just like every other new blogger, I started with zero readers, so what other people thought quickly became less of a concern.

At first I didn't want anyone to read the blog. But the more I wrote, the more I wanted to share with the world. And then all of a sudden I had readers! Complete strangers started to post comments and ask questions. People were looking to me for answers, and I was happy to help. I loved sharing my experiences and advice with others, especially when it came to two of my biggest passions: food and fitness.

Carrots 'N' Cake was born on February 3, 2008. Back then, my posts showed that I was more interested in counting calories than eating wholesome, nutritious foods. In my early posts, I counted every single calorie in all of my meals. I even included calories-burned estimates from my workouts. Boy, how things have changed!

The philosophy behind *Carrots 'N' Cake* was basically "Lose weight, but don't stress out over it." I wanted to lose weight gradually and keep if off. I knew that crash dieting a month before my wedding wouldn't be a good idea. I get stressed-out really easily, so I knew the month before the wedding would be a crazy time for me, and I didn't want to make it worse by thinking constantly about what I was eating and how much I was exercising. I wanted to enjoy my engagement and the wedding planning—things like cake tasting and engagement parties—but I also wanted to drop a few pounds. Finding the balance was what *Carrots 'N' Cake* was all about for me.

When I first started *Carrots 'N' Cake*, I thought counting calories was the way to lose weight. I had lost about twenty pounds a few years earlier by using an online calorie tracker called FitDay.com. Keeping track of the calories that I consumed worked the first time, so I figured it would work again on my blog. Plus, Kath counted her calories, so I thought this was the right way to blog. I mean, she seemed to know what she was doing!

Over time, though, counting calories became really time-consuming, and it seemed my readers were really focused on the numbers. I really wanted my blog to be about living a healthy, balanced life and enjoying the "bad" foods in moderation. Calorie counting seemed to send the wrong message. The calorie counts were important, but eating nutritious foods while enjoying dessert without guilt was the real message I wanted to send. I wanted to show people that I could lose weight and tone up without dieting and obsessing about what I ate. I stopped calorie counting and focused on creating balanced meals with my daily splurges in mind.

Carrots 'N' Cake is all about eating your carrots and having your cake, too. The reason I have been so successful in losing weight and keeping it off is that I've adopted healthy eating habits that have stayed with me for years. Life is all about balance—including enjoying a piece of carrot cake every now and then!

COOKIE FRIDAY

O h, Friday. My favorite day of the entire week. There's just something about Fridays—the slow-moving morning, lingering over coffee with co-workers, the mental vacation that everyone seems to take right around four o'clock. There's also the anticipation of two days off—free to do whatever I want: sleep late, meet up with friends for cocktails, enjoy an indulgent Sunday brunch of French toast and mimosas. What's not to like about Friday?

Friday is also the day I allow myself a splurge. I call it Cookie Friday.

Cookie Friday isn't always about a cookie. It can be any treat I want: a donut, a piece of cake, maybe a pumpkin scone. It doesn't have to be a sweet treat, either. My Cookie Friday can include a plate of cheesy nachos or a bagel as big as my head—with cream cheese. We're talking a splurge of around 500 calories, but it's my treat for the week, so I believe in enjoying it and making it worth my while.

Give a Little, Gain a Little

A 500-calorie splurge might seem pretty huge. Well, it is! Think about the size of my breakfast or even lunch—it's probably around 500 calories, right? But splurging on Cookie Friday is all about balance. I can cut 50 calories from my breakfast by using half as much peanut butter on my English muffin. I can shave another 100 off my lunch by nixing the cheese from my sandwich. It's easy to cut a few calories here and there so I can fully enjoy my Cookie Friday.

And that's important because the real benefit of Cookie Friday is what it does for my psyche. I love sweets, especially baked goods like cookies. Not allowing myself to have them actually makes me sad. A big, freshly baked oatmeal raisin cookie is probably one of my most beloved indulgences. Thinking about my well-deserved splurge all week long helps me say no to the not-so-great splurges—like the store-bought donuts or commercially produced milk chocolate that colleagues share with the office. I could help myself to these treats, but they wouldn't make me as happy as knowing that I saved up my calories for one big, awesome splurge on Friday.

HCLS IS LOOKING FOR
Tech Stop Crew!

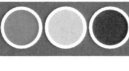

VOLUNTEER THIS SUMMER!

Assist customers with questions about everyday technology. Provide guidance for email, social media, online searches, the use of smart devices, functionality of different Apps, and other technology questions. Volunteers must commit to at least 6 hours of volunteer work (3 sessions) during summer vacation. Volunteers must be in/entering high school and be at least 14 years old on May 1, 2018.

For required qualifications, training, and application, visit hcllibrary.org/support-us/welcome-volunteers/tech-stop-crew-student-volunteer-opportunity

I start my Friday morning like most days: workout, breakfast, blog, commute to office, work until lunchtime. But lunchtime on (Cookie) Friday is different. Friday's lunch is always light: a salad with beans, Greek yogurt with cereal and fruit, or raw veggies with a pita and some hummus. I like to add a lot of volume to lunch in the form of raw vegetables so I fill up my stomach without a lot of added calories.

A cookie really is my favorite Cookie Friday treat. After lunch, I go to Starbucks to order their massive M&M'S cookie and a small coffee with soy milk. Back at the office, I type away on my computer as I catch up on e-mails and enjoy every single bite and sip. I made balanced choices all week, so why not enjoy every minute of my indulgence?

I've always associated baking cookies with special occasions. As the child of a hardworking single mother, I felt somewhat starved for attention at times. I'm not saying that my mom neglected my sister and me in any way—that's not how I grew up at all. But with no financial support from my father, my mom worked two jobs to provide for our family, so she was rarely at home. And, not surprisingly, when she was home, she was often exhausted from working a twelve-hour day.

When my mom had time to spend with my sister and me, food always seemed to be the center of attention. When I was growing up, my family didn't have a lot of money. In fact, we could barely pay the bills, let alone buy any extras, so spending time with Mom meant we'd celebrate with her homemade apple crisp or a box of Duncan Hines brownie mix—a cheap, convenient option for an overworked single mother. The three of us would pitch in and bake together. While we waited for our special treat, we chatted and connected as a family. Enjoying what we had made was always the best part of spending time together, and Mom never limited how much we ate. It was a special occasion, so it was okay to have a big brownie. These splurges became a way for us to bond.

Carrots 'N' Cake might come off as an easy and breezy Web site with a focus on fun and (mostly) healthy living, but in fact, it took me a while to get to this point. Growing up, I never really paid attention to what I ate or how much I exercised. To be honest, I really didn't need to. I never struggled with my weight until I entered high school, when the weight started to creep on. I played sports and took dance classes, so exercise kept my weight steady, but I ate a lot of junk food. Kraft macaroni and cheese, ramen noodles, and Betty Crocker brownies were staples in my diet.

In high school, I'd eat two cinnamon Pop-Tarts for breakfast, then go through the entire school day and a two-hour soccer practice, not eating again until dinnertime. No wonder I binged on unhealthy foods as soon as I got home—I hadn't eaten all day! I remember many nights after a game or long practice, I'd come home tired and cranky, wolf down whatever my mother made for dinner, and then mix up a batch of brownies (or cookies) and eat at least half of the batch. It would be late by the time I started my homework or began studying for an exam, so I'd stay up well into the night munching on baked goods to deal with my anxiety. I've always been a type A person, especially when it came to making good grades, and food continued to be my go-to method for dealing with the stress and anxiety that went with being graded. In college, I'd always have a bag of candy or some cookies by my side when I studied. And I still remember one finals week when I finished off an entire box of cereal over the course of a night as I stayed up cramming for back-to-back finals the next day.

My mom also used sweet treats as a way to celebrate special occasions and achievements in our lives. On Christmas morning, one of our family traditions is to bake Pillsbury Cinnamon Rolls, the ones that are covered with sticky white frosting. We have these for breakfast before we open our gifts. When I was growing up, for less than three dollars the three of us could share this indulgent breakfast without breaking the bank. Our family's financial situation has changed, but we still keep this Christmas morning tradition—with a few tweaks. Nowadays, Mom buys freshly squeezed orange juice and my sister and I bring fresh fruit salad to enjoy along with our cinnamon buns. We've learned a few things about nutrition!

After years of struggling with overeating as a way to relieve stress, I eventually acknowledged it as an issue. It didn't happen overnight, though. There was a lot of trial and error and figuring out what worked best for me. Cookie Friday is like a celebration for me—a reward for working hard all week in the office and making good choices for living a healthy lifestyle.

Here Are a Few Delicious Ways to Enjoy Cookie Friday:

BANANA OATMEAL CHIP COOKIES

These cookies taste way too delectable to be good for you—but they really are as nutritious as they are delicious. Superstar ingredients include ground flaxseed meal, banana, soy milk, agave nectar, whole wheat flour, walnuts, and canola oil. Sounds like an all-star cast to me! Added bonus: these cookies are vegan.

1/2 cup whole wheat flour

1 cup old-fashioned oats

1/2 teaspoon baking powder

1/2 teaspoon baking soda

1/4 teaspoon ground cinnamon

1 tablespoon ground flaxseed meal

1/4 cup agave nectar (or honey)

1/4 cup soy milk

1/2 teaspoon vanilla extract

1 tablespoon canola oil

1 ripe banana

1/2 cup chocolate chips

1/4 cup chopped walnuts (optional)

Preheat the oven to 350°F and grease a large baking sheet. Combine all the ingredients in a large bowl and mix well until dough is blended evenly.

Using a tablespoon, portion the dough onto the baking sheet, spacing the cookies about 1 to 2 inches apart. Bake for 10 to 12 minutes, until golden brown. Remove cookies from baking sheet and allow to cool on wire rack. Enjoy!

MAKES ABOUT 25 COOKIES

"HEALTHIER" BLONDIES

Who doesn't love blondies? Most of us remember them as the star of grammar school bake sales. These are every bit as good, but they're the grown-up version, made with canned pumpkin and soy milk for added moisture and flavor.

1 cup all-purpose flour

1 cup brown sugar

1/4 cup canola oil

1/3 cup canned pumpkin

1 tablespoon molasses

2 teaspoons vanilla extract

1/2 teaspoon baking soda

1/4 cup vanilla soy milk

1 cup chocolate chips

1/4 cup chopped walnuts

Preheat the oven to 325°F, and spray an 8-inch square baking pan with nonstick cooking spray. In a large bowl, combine all ingredients and mix until smooth. Spread batter in prepared baking pan and bake for 25 to 30 minutes, until a wooden pick (or knife) inserted near the center comes out clean. Let blondies cool completely in baking pan before cutting.

MAKES 12 BLONDIES

PEANUT BUTTER COOKIES

I have a weakness for peanut butter cookies, and once in a while I just have to have them—on a Friday, of course. Since the batter needs to chill, sometimes I whip up the batter the night before and bake the cookies the next day.

11/4 cups sifted all-purpose flour

3/4 teaspoon baking soda

1/2 teaspoon baking powder

1/4 teaspoon salt

1/2 cup (1 stick) butter, softened

1/2 cup chunky-style peanut butter

1/2 cup granulated sugar

1/2 cup firmly packed light brown sugar

1 egg

Combine the flour, baking soda, baking powder, and salt in a sifter, mix well, and sift onto a sheet of waxed paper. Combine the butter and peanut butter in a large bowl and beat with an electric mixer until blended. Gradually add the granulated sugar and brown sugar and beat until light and fluffy. Beat in the egg. Add the flour mixture and beat at low speed until well combined. Cover and refrigerate until well chilled, about 1 hour.

Preheat the oven to 350°F and line baking sheets with parchment paper. Shape the dough into ¾-inch balls and place 2 inches apart on the prepared sheets. Flatten with a fork, making a crisscross pattern on each cookie. Bake until lightly browned, about 6 minutes. Cool on the sheets for a few minutes, then transfer to wire racks to cool completely.

MAKES ABOUT 50 SMALL COOKIES

PUMPKIN SPICE COOKIES

If you think about pumpkin muffin tops packed with lots of walnuts and raisins, well, you get the idea. I can't tell you how many times I've made these for my Cookie Friday treat.

     1 cup spelt flour
     1 cup canned pumpkin
     4 tablespoons softened butter
    1/2 cup packed brown sugar
    1/4 cup ground flaxseed meal
    1/2 teaspoon ground cinnamon
    1/4 teaspoon grated nutmeg
    1/4 teaspoon ground ginger
    1/2 cup chopped walnuts
    1/2 cup raisins

Preheat the oven to 350°F. and grease a baking sheet. Combine all the ingredients in a large bowl and mix well. Drop the dough in 8 equal mounds onto the prepared baking sheet, and bake until the cookies start to brown, about 25 to 30 minutes. Let the cookies cool before serving.

MAKES 8 LARGE COOKIES

DATE NIGHT

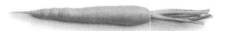

I love Date Night. Date Night is an opportunity for my husband, Mal, and me to leave the responsibilities of life behind and just enjoy each other's company—sort of like we did when we were dating. Our lives are so busy that sometimes I think we take each other for granted, so when we have the time—and don't have plans with friends— a Date Night is a way to connect and to appreciate our time together as a couple.

Mal and I always have a blast on Date Night. We build the anticipation by talking about it from the time we wake up that morning. We start talking about Date Night at breakfast: where we'll go for dinner, whether we'll get dessert or not, and what we'll wear. And we ask the question, "Are you excited for Date Night?" over and over again, all day long. If you hung out with us on Saturday afternoon, you'd think it was really annoying, but we're goofy like that.

Young Love

Mal and I have a long history of Date Nights. We've known each other since we were kids (my sister and Mal have been friends since kindergarten), and we even dated in high school. That caused a minor scandal in our small town, since Mal was a freshman and I was a senior. I was casually dating one of his friends at the time, but the more Mal and I hung out, the more the attraction grew. Soon, we found ourselves hanging out after school and making plans to get together on the weekend. Before we knew it, we were boyfriend and girlfriend and dated for about six months before I went off to college.

Dating Mal has always been easy. Even as teenagers, we seemed to have this weird connection. From our first date, which was actually a double date with another couple, I've always felt at ease with him. We never really had those awkward moments that most new couples have when they first start dating. Of course, we've both done plenty of embarrassing things in our relationship, but it's easy to laugh them off and move on. Our relationship actually thrives on the two of us laughing with (and at) each other. Thank goodness we both have a good sense of humor! I think there would be a lot of hurt feelings otherwise.

Mal and I stayed in touch over the years between high school and college. We'd get together for coffee or lunch anytime we were both home from school. We had other relationships and we each did our own thing, but we always remained in contact.

The Wednesday before Thanksgiving 2003, Mal was home from college and I was working at Boston College in the Undergraduate Admissions Office. I was already in vacation mode and ready to have a few days off, so I took a break from work and chatted online with some of my friends. While I was chatting away, Mal sent me a message and asked if I was free the following weekend to get together. I already had plans to attend a friend's birthday party at a bowling alley in the city, so I invited him along.

Sparks Flew

A few days later, Mal drove into the city and met me at my apartment. I still remember opening the door and seeing his face for the first time in a couple of years. We were both single at the time, and the sparks flew right from the beginning of our night. We had a blast bowling with my friends. There was a lot of laughing and cracking jokes, like old times. It felt like we hadn't lost any time at all.

Mal was midway through the first semester of his junior year of college, so he went back to school right after Thanksgiving break. We hadn't established any sort of relationship before he left—I mean, we hung out one night—but we said we'd be in touch. We were both interested in pursuing something, but neither of us was sure about a long-distance relationship. Plus, Mal was enjoying

his single life at college and I was enjoying mine in Boston.
Even though we had some serious chemistry, a relationship
wasn't on our minds in the beginning.

A few weeks passed before Mal was home again for
Christmas break. We had chatted on the phone maybe two
or three times during the time he was back at school. As
soon as he was home at his parents' house, though, we made
plans to get together—and we hung out pretty much every
night while he was home. When he headed back to school
in early January, we talked about the prospect of a relationship. We already knew each other pretty well, so falling into
a relationship again was really easy. The long-distance part
of the relationship was a lot more difficult, but somehow we
managed. A year and a half later, Mal was living in Boston,
and the rest is history!

On our wedding day, my father-in-law made a toast at
the reception. He said a number of heartfelt things about
us as individuals and as a couple, including that Mal and I
complement each other perfectly. Well, technically, he said
that we complement one another's individual neuroses very
well, but we knew what he meant!

Even though Mal and I are both uptight, generally
high-strung, type A people, we make it work. I stress about
things that he could care less about, and vice versa. For
instance, as soon as I see the laundry hamper starting to
get full, I need to start washing a load, while he wouldn't
think twice about it. Similarly, he has to make the bed
every morning, while I usually leave the bedding a mess
until I climb into it to sleep again. We seem to balance
each other out.

On the food front, we also complement each other nicely. When it comes to cupcakes, I love the frosting top, while he would much rather eat the cakey bottom. It works out great! All joking aside, when it comes to eating, we really do balance each other out. I have been a healthy influence on him when it comes to eating more nutritious foods, and he has helped me try new foods and lighten up on my choices. Before Mal, I would have never eaten a hot dog, but now when a summer barbecue or ball game rolls around, I am more than happy to indulge in one. On the other hand, Mal would have never eaten oatmeal for breakfast, and now he requests that I make it for him some mornings. (He's pretty much addicted to oatmeal, like I am, now.)

Pop-Tarts to Oatmeal

Monday through Friday, I wake up with Mal at six o'clock, even though I don't need to be at work for three more hours. It's not because I'm trying to squeeze in a workout or a sunrise yoga session—it's because I enjoy making him breakfast. Usually I make us a big batch of banana oatmeal and add all the fixings—wheat berries, almonds, chia seeds, and a scoop of peanut butter. Being a grown man, Mal is more than capable of cooking himself a healthy breakfast, but I really enjoy helping him start his day off on the right foot. Plus, eating breakfast together is easily my favorite part of the day. We watch *SportsCenter* and drink our iced coffees on the couch. We talk about the upcoming week and what is on the agenda for the day. It's a nice way to start the day together.

I never considered myself a nurturing person until I started cooking for my husband. In fact, the act of cooking sort of scared me—mostly because I was terrible at it! Growing up, I never really learned to cook. Since Mom was a single parent, the majority of our meals were quick and easy convenience meals. I ate Pop-Tarts for breakfast, boxed mac 'n' cheese for lunch, and microwavable meals for dinner—which, of course, weren't the most nutritious foods to eat. But in my mother's defense, she managed to provide for my sister and me, and I think my sister and I were just happy to have her home with us! We almost never complained about what Mom made for dinner, and if we did, her response was always the same: "I'm not running a restaurant." She made the effort to put something on the table, which we always appreciated.

Mom planted the seed that even if you're short on time, sitting down for a meal—any meal—is a form of bonding. Over the years I've changed the way that I eat, and I've realized just how much food is love. I used to focus on low-calorie and low-fat foods—typically ones made with artificial ingredients—but I soon learned that they don't make me feel as good as "real" food does. For instance, a snack of an apple with lots of fiber and nutrients satisfies me much more than a couple of apple-cinnamon rice cakes. Choosing real foods over fake ones makes me feel like I am choosing to treat my body right. Similarly, picking high-quality ingredients for my meals also makes me feel like I am taking good care of myself—and now my husband, too.

A Taste for Adventure

More than once while growing up, I remember trying something that I didn't think I would like and realizing it was pretty good. Today, my sister and I are the least picky eaters you will ever meet. We'll eat anything! Thankfully, my husband is adventurous when it comes to food, too. There are a few foods he doesn't like—mostly things that are "squishy," like eggplant and squash—but otherwise, he'll pretty much eat anything. So dining out is easy for us. We love trying new places, and both of us can always find something on the menu that sounds appetizing.

One night we dined at a Spanish tapas restaurant in the South End of Boston; we ordered cow tongue and bone marrow among other more "traditional" tapas just because we were in the mood to try something new and different. When it comes to dining out, my husband doesn't necessarily encourage me to try new foods, but he's always on board when I suggest it. I'm definitely the more adventurous eater of the two.

As a blogger, I am often contacted by restaurants to dine out at their establishments. Usually, someone who does public relations for the restaurant contacts me, but other times, it's an owner or a chef. Typically, I am asked to share my dining experience on *Carrots 'N' Cake* in exchange for a free meal. My husband is often invited, too, so it's a nice way for us to enjoy our time together without spending a lot of money. Plus, I enjoy writing restaurant reviews, and my readers typically like reading them.

Planning for Indulgence

Tonight's Date Night would be dinner at an upscale Italian restaurant. Mal and I had been invited as guests of the owners. With an indulgent meal on the horizon, I start

making balanced eating choices as soon as I wake up. I can't
fully enjoy a meal out if I don't make healthy decisions all
day long.

I start with a healthy (and relatively low-calorie) bowl
of stove-top oatmeal with wheat berries (recipe on page 23).
It's a combination of carbs, protein, and healthy fats that
keeps me full all morning. Plus, the mushy bowl of oatmeal
is warm, filling, and satisfying; I don't even think about food
again for hours.

After I eat breakfast, I usually take our dog, Murphy,
for a thirty-minute walk around the neighborhood. It's a
great way to start the day with a little activity and a happy
pug face. Plus, the walk helps me digest my food a bit. Once
Murphy and I return from our walk, I head straight to
my computer to blog. It takes me anywhere from thirty
to sixty minutes to create a typical breakfast post, which
is usually just long enough for me to digest my food. Once
dog walking and blogging is complete, it's time to break a
sweat!

Burn Baby Burn

If I'm going to splurge, I need to get a head start on
burning up those extra calories! I don't do this workout
every Saturday morning, but I like to do a similar-style
workout with lots of cardio—usually intervals—so I get a
serious calorie burn. It makes me feel better about indulging
later in the day.

TREADMILL WORKOUT

Total time: *45 minutes*

- Walk at 4.0 mph at 7.5 incline for 4 minutes
- Jog at 6.5 mph at 1.0 incline for 5 minutes
- Repeat walk and jog 2 times
- Jog at 6.5 mph at 2.0 incline for 3 minutes
- Run at 7.0 mph at 1.0 incline for 3 minutes
- Sprint at 8.0 mph at 1.0 incline for 1 minute
- Jog at 6.0 mph at 1.0 incline for 1 minute
- Sprint at 8.0 mph at 1.0 incline for 1 minute
- Run at 7.0 mph at 1.0 incline for 1 minute
- Jog at 6.5 mph at 1.0 incline for 3 minutes
- Walk (cool down) for 5 minutes

I arrive home sweaty, exhausted, and hungry! Breakfast did a great job holding off my hunger for many hours, but now that I've burned through my morning bowl of oats, it's time to refuel. Even though a big splurge is planned for later in the day, I don't skip any meals. First of all, I like to eat, but also, being hungry makes me cranky, and I don't want to be starving by the time we get to the restaurant. My easy Mediterranean salad (recipe on page 22) is hearty and satisfying, yet not too heavy. It's just light enough to bank some of my calories, but it has enough staying power to hold me over until dinnertime. I remind myself that reviewing the restaurant allows us to order anything off the menu we want, so it isn't tough to save up my calories that afternoon.

Mal and I have been looking forward to Date Night all day long, so when it comes time to get ready for our big night out, we make sure to make it an event. While we shower, dress, and make ourselves presentable, we play some rocking music in our apartment. Michael Jackson, Oasis, and Journey put us in a good mood for a fun night.

As much as I love getting dressed up for a night out, my husband loves it even more. Sometimes he spends more time thinking about what to wear than I do! I love that he takes the time to consider how he looks on our special nights out.

I also make an effort to look nice on our Date Nights. Usually, I wear something formfitting, which is, of course, for my husband, but also for me. Mal likes it when I show off my body a little bit, and so do I, but I also wear tight jeans or pants to help me practice moderation at dinner. It's so easy for me to overdo it at restaurants; wearing clothing that is a little snug is a constant reminder of when to stop.

Hunger pains aren't typically a problem for me because I like to eat every few hours to keep my hunger at bay and my blood sugar steady. However, there are times when I'm unable to eat or I forget to eat until it's too late and my stomach is growling like crazy. I call these times "emergency situations" because I feel like I need to eat ASAP or I start to get cranky—and no one wants to be around me when I am cranky! At the same time, if I know a big meal or special night out, like Date Night, is on the agenda in the next two or three hours, I can usually wait to eat something. If it's more than three hours, I *need* to eat a snack to hold me over. The two- to three-hour window is usually my max for waiting to eat if I am hungry. Any longer, and I know I will go overboard when faced with delicious food. Now, when dinnertime rolls around, my stomach starts growling—loudly! I haven't eaten since lunch.

Mal and I usually enjoy a cocktail at home before we go out to dinner on Date Night. Spending time together in the comfort of our own home is a nice way to connect and focus on each other before the date even begins—and less expensive than ordering a drink in a restaurant, too. Since we are receiving dinner for free tonight—and I'm hungry!—we opt to skip the predinner cocktail and head right out.

The restaurant is about a thirty-minute drive outside the city, so by the time we arrive, I am more than ready to splurge. But while I love a good restaurant meal, I don't let myself get carried away. Instead of immediately grabbing a roll from the bread basket, I make a mental game plan for dinner.

Here's My Thought Process:

First, I assess the menu. What are my meal options? Do the meals come with a side salad? The pasta dishes are probably a huge portion. I'm starving, but would I be better off ordering an appetizer instead of an entrée? Then, I figure out what I'm in the mood to eat. Pasta? Fish? Chicken? Perhaps something new and different?

This might seem like a lot of work (and obsessing), but it's really not. It doesn't take me that long to decide what I want. I know I'm going to indulge myself, but I want to do it in the right way.

As it happens, the chef prepares a tasting menu for us, which makes my decision for me. It also forces me to alter my game plan for the evening. I ask our waiter how many courses will be served. His response: seven! Oh boy. This means I need to pace myself!

I start by nixing the bread basket. If I have seven courses of authentic Italian cuisine ahead of me, I do not need to waste my calories on bread. Over the course of the meal, I serve myself small portions of everything—no more than three or four bites. I do go back for seconds of the homemade egg pasta, which is out of this world! I also do some damage on dessert, but I had paced myself and practiced some self-control for the majority of the meal, so it was okay to fully enjoy dessert. Mal and I eat the whole thing!

I probably ate more calories than I usually would at a normal dinner at home, but I planned for my meal the right way—by saving up calories and appetite. And the best part about the evening was that I enjoyed myself 100 percent guilt free. I didn't have to think twice about enjoying dessert!

Helpful Hint: Practice the two-out-of-three rule when dining out. Have a dinner roll and a martini, but skip dessert. If you really want dessert and a glass of wine, don't bother with a dinner roll. Pick two out of three and enjoy. Just don't have them all!

To recap: Turn the page for my go-to breakfast and lunch recipes leading up to my big-splurge Date Nights out:

EASY MEDITERRANEAN SALAD

Crumbled feta adds a bit of protein to this yummy salad. I like to
serve mine over a bed of greens for some added volume.

---

3 Yukon gold potatoes, diced

1/4 cup plus two tablespoons olive oil

Salt

1 red bell pepper, seeded and diced

1 small Vidalia onion, diced

1/2 cup pitted Kalamata olives

1 (6-ounce) jar marinated artichoke hearts, drained and
   chopped

1/2 cup diced feta cheese

2 tomatoes, diced

1/4 cup balsamic vinegar

Freshly ground pepper

Preheat the oven to 450°F.

Place the potatoes in a large mixing bowl. Drizzle with 1 tablespoon olive oil, sprinkle with salt, and toss to coat. Transfer
the potatoes to a shallow roasting pan, and roast for 15 to
20 minutes or until golden brown.

Meanwhile, heat 1 tablespoon olive oil in a small frying pan,
add the bell pepper, and sauté until softened.

In a large mixing bowl, combine the onion, olives, artichoke
hearts, feta, tomatoes, ¼ cup olive oil, the balsamic vinegar,
and salt and pepper. When the potatoes and peppers are

cooked, add them to the bowl, and mix well. Allow to cool in the refrigerator for about an hour. Serve cold over a bed of your favorite greens, if desired, and enjoy!

MAKES 4 SERVINGS

STOVE-TOP OATMEAL
WITH WHEAT BERRIES

Hearty, filling, and satisfying, this little breakfast keeps me full all morning long, and I can whip it up in minutes.

1/2 cup old-fashioned oats

1 banana, sliced

2 tablespoons cooked berries (see page 38)

1 tablespoon ground flaxseed meal

1 cup soy milk

1 tablespoon peanut butter

Combine all ingredients, except the peanut butter, in a pot on the stove top. Cook oatmeal over medium heat until it thickens. Pour oatmeal into a bowl and add the peanut butter. Serve hot.

MAKES 1 SERVING

STRENGTH TRAINING IS NOT EXTRA CREDIT

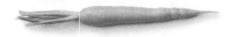

It's Sunday morning. The sun is shining. The birds are chirping. I am ready to start the day. I tackle my usual routine—breakfast (oatmeal) and blogging (about oatmeal)—and then it's time to tackle my to-do list. For me, Sunday is not a day of rest!

First Task: Exercise

Sunday mornings are a great time to devote to strength training. Typically, the gym is empty and quiet. There's plenty of space to spread out, I don't have to wait my turn for any of the equipment, and I don't have to rush through my workout. If I want to use a bench for chest press, I don't have to wait until someone else finishes or rearrange my workout to make sure that I fit it in. I love having my pick of the best equipment, too. I get my favorite kind of dumbbells and use the elliptical right in front of the television with my favorite shows on Bravo—not the one that continuously plays CNN.

I almost always wake up sore on Monday morning—a feeling that I love after working hard the day before. On Sunday mornings, I take my time with strength training. I listen to my iPod, concentrate, and make sure I get the best workout possible. It's easier to focus when I don't feel self-conscious about weight lifting. Those meathead weight lifters aren't usually at the gym on Sunday morning to intimidate me. There's been more than one time that I've skipped part of my routine because I felt embarrassed with those guys hanging around.

Things I hate about strength training:
the boredom
crowded gyms
feeling self-conscious around meatheads

Things I love about strength training:
the results
feeling strong and powerful
the *results*

For a long time, I halfheartedly tried to add strength training to my workout, but I really didn't know what to do and I found it boring. Not surprisingly, I never got into a consistent routine. I basically thought that a little weight lifting was better than none! After a run on the treadmill, for instance, I'd be huffing and puffing. When I strength trained, I'd often finish a workout feeling like I hadn't done much work. Without challenging my muscles by lifting enough weight, I wasn't doing myself any favors.

I really got into strength training around the same time that I started *Carrots 'N' Cake*. I had been blogging for a few weeks and recording my workouts, but when I looked back I realized that I hadn't included even a mention of strength training. It wasn't long before I was Googling strength-training programs that would help me shape up for my wedding. I had always been a fan of cardio, but with only a few more months to go, I knew that I needed to step it up with some weights if I wanted to look good in my wedding dress.

Bridal Bootcamp

I found a free twelve-week Bridal Bootcamp workout online that I stuck to religiously in the weeks up to my wedding. The program required that I complete cardio and strength-training workouts five times a week. I thought it seemed like a lot of strength training, but I was determined to shape up and look great on my wedding day, so I followed the program almost exactly.

There were days when I made some changes, like when I didn't have time for a full strength-training workout and did a shorter cardio workout instead. I did all of the workouts during their assigned week, but they weren't always in the same order as the program instructed.

During those twelve weeks, I learned a lot about strength training—and about myself. The program made me work hard each and every day at the gym, which was something that I slacked off on every now and then. I was putting my time in, but I wasn't seeing results. It was so easy to grab a magazine and zone out on the elliptical. Sure, I was burning some calories, but for the amount of time I was spending casually peddling along, I could have been working my body a lot harder. Strength training showed me that if I wanted to see results, I needed to work hard and be consistent.

Suddenly, Muscles

About six weeks passed before I started to see real results. Suddenly, I noticed muscles I never knew I had. My shoulders looked tight and toned, and my biceps started to bulge (at least I thought so). Seeing results also kept me motivated to add regular strength-training workouts to my weekly routine at the gym. Weight lifting made me feel strong, too. I love the feeling of fatigued muscles after a tough workout. And I love the soreness I feel the day after a good workout—it's a constant reminder of how hard I work.

The Bridal Bootcamp workout made me realize for the first time ever that strength training really makes a difference. I always knew that I *should* strength train, but I always thought it was boring, so I never consistently did it. In twelve weeks, using this workout, I started to see changes in my body. My arms and legs got *thinner* and more toned. I was worried about bulking up, but it never happened. I finally got the body I wanted and realized that it didn't require hours and hours of cardio.

Today, I still incorporate quite a bit of strength training into my weekly workouts. I typically take two to three Body Pump classes each week, which work all of my major muscle groups in a fifty-five-minute class. I'm sort of obsessed with Body Pump, especially how it makes me feel and what it does to the shape of my body. For instance, the summer after I began Body Pump was the first summer in a long time that all of my shorts and skirts fit me after a long winter. I had been consistently attending Body Pump classes for nearly a year, which made all the difference.

Having a Game Plan

Today, I arrive at the gym with a "plan of attack." I've written down my strength-training workout for the day: a 45-minute full-body workout that utilizes free weights as well as machines. Writing down my strength-training workout keeps me focused on the task at hand. If I don't record my workout before I start lifting weights, I end up wandering aimlessly around the weight room, doing a set of exercises and working different muscles here or there. My routine becomes random, so I don't get as good a workout. Plus, if I don't have a game plan for my workout, it's easy to just quit halfway through. I hate starting something and not finishing it, so I almost never leave a planned workout unfinished.

On Sunday morning at the gym, I warm up for 10 minutes by walking on the treadmill, and then I get to it! This is not a beginner's workout. It took me six to eight months to build up to this point, and looking back, I see how much stronger I am now.

Chest fly with dumbbells: 15 reps, 3 sets, 12 pounds

Single-arm dumbbell rows: 15 reps, 3 sets, 12 pounds

Dumbbell shoulder press: 15 reps, 3 sets, 12 pounds

Seated dumbbell biceps curl: 15 reps, 3 sets, 10 pounds

Overhead triceps extension: 15 reps, 3 sets, 12 pounds

Squats: 15 reps, 3 sets, 15 pounds

Calf raises: 15 reps, 3 sets, body weight

Plank pose: 60 seconds, 3 sets, body weight

If you're just starting out, here's a good routine to get you going—you'll hurt (no pain, no gain!), but you won't hurt yourself.

Chest fly with dumbbells: 10 reps, 2 sets, 8 pounds

Single-arm dumbbell rows: 10 reps, 2 sets, 8 pounds

Dumbbell shoulder press: 10 reps, 2 sets, 5 pounds

Seated dumbbell biceps curl: 10 reps, 2 sets, 5 pounds

Overhead triceps extension: 10 reps, 2 sets, 5 pounds

Squats: 10 reps, 2 sets, 10 pounds

Calf raises: 10 reps, 2 sets, body weight

Plank pose: 30 seconds, 2 sets, body weight

While lifting, I listen to classic rock. I need this type of motivation to keep myself moving. No matter what anyone says, I still think weight lifting is boring. I do it because it makes my body look good, but if I didn't get the results that I do from it, I probably wouldn't devote so much time and energy to it. I also focus on how my muscles look while I am strength training. Seeing my muscles moving and shaping up provides constant positive reinforcement and pushes me to work hard.

The key to this workout is not to rest more than 20 seconds between exercises to make sure that I am working my muscles to fatigue. For example, on the leg-press machine, I drop to 90 pounds on the last set because my quads and glutes are burning by then! I want to push myself hard, but I know when it's time to drop weight. Recording my workouts and checking each exercise off my list gives me the stick-with-it attitude that helps push me through my workout.

I strength train at least three times per week in order to see continuous results in my abilities and body. A trainer once told me, "Strength train once a week to maintain, twice to see improvements, and three times to see results," so now I really make it a point to do a full-body (upper- and lower-body exercises) strength-training workout three times a week. For convenience, I sometimes break my full-body workout into separate upper- and lower-body strength-training workouts—mostly because I am crunched for time and want to fit in some cardio at the gym, too. I rarely spend more than an hour at the gym on any given day, with half of my workout devoted to strength training and the other half devoted to cardio.

The way I see it, strength training gives me results, but cardio keeps me sane—it's so good for my mental health. Despite the amount of physical energy required for cardio-vascular exercise, it actually calms me. A long run after a rough day at the office always makes me feel a million times less stressed. Even a quickie elliptical workout with a trashy celebrity gossip magazine puts me in a better mood. There's just something about breaking a sweat that totally puts me in a better mind-set.

Helpful Hint: If you're intimidated by strength training, try a group exercise class like Body Pump. Body Pump was the perfect opportunity for me to learn the basics of weight lifting. Typically, these classes challenge all of your major muscle groups using a weighted bar, dumbbells, or resistance bands, or some combination of the three.

POST-WORKOUT
SWEET POTATO SMOOTHIE

I usually drink this smoothie for breakfast or lunch after a work-out as a way to refuel. All the different nutrients plus the protein help rebuild my muscles. Bonus: this smoothie is really filling and keeps me full until my next meal.

1/2 cup mashed sweet potato

1 ripe banana

1/4 cup nonfat plain Greek yogurt

1/4 cup vanilla soy milk

1 tablespoon hemp (or whey) protein

1 tablespoon agave nectar (or honey)

1/2 teaspoon vanilla extract

1/2 teaspoon ground cinnamon

1/2 cup ice

Dash of grated nutmeg

Combine all the ingredients in a blender and puree until smooth. Serve in a tall glass, preferably with a stainless-steel straw.

MAKES 1 SMOOTHIE

OUT OF SIGHT, OUT OF MIND

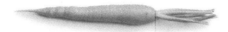

I have my own cabinet in our kitchen. Inside is all of the "health" food that I like to eat—Lärabars, almond butter, smoothie powders. They're all in one place, so I don't forget about the healthy foods available in my kitchen. They're also in a special place separate from what my husband is "allowed" to eat. It's not that I don't like to share, but if I don't declare some of this food off-limits, he eats it all before I even have a bite. More important, however, is that when they're all in one place that is easily within view, I don't forget about them.

It's Monday morning. I just returned home from the gym, and now it's time to make breakfast. I go to my special cabinet and scan my options—packets of Barney Butter, dried apricots, Scharffen Berger dark chocolate, and pistachios—but nothing grabs my attention. I'm not in the mood for any of those foods, so I start digging a little deeper into my cabinet.

I'm not necessarily a messy person, but I could definitely be more organized when it comes to my personal food cabinet. Companies often send me free samples of different food items to try, and sometimes they pile up before I have a chance to use them. As I dig through the random mix of healthy options, a tiny rolled bag of wheat berries falls onto the countertop.

Wheat berries! Immediately, I want to cook up a batch right away. I love wheat berries. How could I have forgotten about them for so many weeks?

Eureka! Clear Containers

There's a lot of truth behind the saying "out of sight, out of mind." Of course, it applies to a box of store-bought cookies or bag of potato chips, but have I ever thought about it related to nutritious foods? Take wheat berries, for example. When I have a supply of wheat berries in my refrigerator, I see them almost every time I open the door. Seeing wheat berries in a clear container is a constant reminder to add them to my morning bowl of oats, an afternoon cup of soup, and a dinner salad.

This type of thinking extends to other healthy foods as well, which is why I keep my kitchen well stocked with all of my favorite nutritious items. In order to have plenty of easily accessible food in our home, Mal and I make it a point to go grocery shopping every week. If we don't, there's a danger that we'd end up ordering takeout or going out to a restaurant for a meal, which ends up being an expensive and sometimes high-calorie habit.

Watching Our Pennies

Of course I love having lots of healthy foods around, but it's also another response to food that has its roots in my childhood. There were times growing up when my mother worried whether she could afford to pay the grocery bill each week. Like typical kids, my sister and I always begged for the newest food product on the market—Lunchables, Dunkaroos, and the like—but Mom always turned us down. Why spend three dollars on Lunchables when she could buy a whole box of crackers for the same amount? Food purchases in our house came down to value for the dollar. Luckily, Little Debbie Snacks were a dollar for a box of ten. They were packed with trans fats, but we loved 'em!

Mom would send my sister and me on "shopping adventures"; we'd go up and down the aisles of the grocery store looking for the products that matched our coupons. It kept us busy while she shopped, but it also taught me how to buy groceries on a budget at an early age. Today, I never go grocery shopping without a stack of coupons, and usually I use quite a few. I can't help but look for the best deal possible—and why not? Eating healthy doesn't have to be expensive.

By Monday our kitchen is completely stocked with food for the week, and I have a ton of healthy options for breakfast. Oatmeal is typically my go-to breakfast, so I could make my favorite stove-top version with some ground flaxseed meal and some wheat berries (recipe on page 22). Some days, however, I decide to make my Warm Carrot Cake–Wheat Berry Cereal (see page 39).

I love wheat berries. They're a very satisfying grain with a slightly nutty flavor and a hearty, chewy texture. I used to eat them all the time; I'd mix them into oatmeal, toss them into salads, and add them to soups and even yogurt. Wheat berries were a delicious and nutritious part of my diet—and then a few months went by when I basically forgot that they existed. This can easily happen with other health foods when I don't take the time to make them easily accessible. Soon, convenience items and packaged foods creep their way into my diet. Fresh vegetables are replaced by artificial "veggie" chips, and whole grains are replaced by muffins as big as my head.

Visibility is Key

To make sure I don't forget about the wheat berries I just cooked, I store them in clear plastic containers. Since I try to bring my lunch to work each day, it's a great way to remember exactly what I have on hand, and my lunch is already easily transportable. I also place healthy pantry items, like oats, beans, and peanut butter, at eye level on easy-to-reach shelves in my cupboard. By giving these foods the most visibility, I'm more likely to reach for them. I store tempting treats—a bag of potato chips, cookies, or chocolate—where I can't see them, like in a top cupboard or a drawer in my fridge. Sometimes I even forget that they're there!

Helpful Hint: Instead of keeping fresh fruits and veggies in the crisper drawers in the refrigerator where I can't see them, I put my produce in a big, clear container on the top shelf. Whenever I open the refrigerator, it's the first thing I see. However, I don't ignore those crisper drawers completely. I keep my meats and cheeses as well as my chocolate chip stash there, so I'm less likely to choose them as a snack. Again, out of sight, out of mind.

Another Helpful Hint: I bought a beautiful fruit bowl to display on my kitchen counter, and I keep it stocked with plenty of seasonal produce. The bowl is a constant reminder to incorporate these foods into my diet, and the vibrant colors are a gorgeous addition to my kitchen.

HOW TO COOK WHEAT BERRIES

There are two methods that can be used to prepare wheat berries: the soaking and sprouting method; and the boiling method. I suggest that you try both to see which you prefer. The soaking and sprouting method will produce a softer consistency; the straight boiling method produces a chewier texture, which I prefer.

SOAKING AND SPROUTING METHOD

The first time I made wheat berries, I used the soaking method. They came out great, but the whole process took a lot longer than I expected.

1 cup uncooked wheat berries

Soak the wheat berries in water overnight. The next morning, simmer them on the stove top until chewy, about 45 minutes. (These wheat berries will not keep very long, so eat them as soon as possible.)

MAKES 4 SERVINGS

BOILING METHOD

The second time I prepared wheat berries, I used the boiling method.

1/2 cup uncooked wheat berries

Add the wheat berries to a pot and cover them with water. Bring to a boil, and then simmer until chewy, about 45 minutes.

Drain the wheat berries. (These wheat berries can be stored in a plastic container in the refrigerator for up to 10 days.)

MAKES 2 SERVINGS

WARM CARROT CAKE– WHEAT BERRY CEREAL

You can add wheat berries to just about anything, but they really shine in this breakfast combination. It's a healthy, hearty way to start a cold winter morning.

1/4 cup old-fashioned rolled oats

1/2 cup vanilla soy milk

1/4 cup cooked wheat berries

1/4 cup shredded carrot

1 tablespoon raisins

1 tablespoon chopped walnuts

1 teaspoon brown sugar

1/4 teaspoon ground cinnamon

1/8 teaspoon ground ginger

Combine all ingredients in a pot on the stove top. Bring to a boil, then turn the heat to medium. Cook oatmeal over medium heat until it thickens. Pour into a bowl. Serve hot.

MAKES 1 SERVING

HOMEMADE GRANOLA AND YOGURT

Oats and nuts are so good for you, and making your own granola is so easy. Use just a few tablespoons of this granola mixture over yogurt and you'll have enough for an entire week.

1 cup dry oats

1/2 cup almonds (or your favorite nut)

1/3 cup shredded coconut

1/4 cup pumpkin seeds or sesame seeds

1 tablespoon ground flaxseed meal

3 tablespoons agave nectar

1 tablespoon canola oil

Shake of ground cinnamon

1/3 cup raisins

Preheat the oven to 350°F. Add everything except the raisins to a large bowl and stir well until the agave nectar and canola oil are fully mixed in (it'll start to get a little clumpy). Spray a baking pan with nonstick cooking spray, and spread the granola out in the pan. Bake for 15 to 18 minutes, stirring occasionally. Remove granola from oven and mix in raisins. Allow to cool before serving. Store in an airtight container.

MAKES ABOUT 2 CUPS

POMEGRANATE APPLE CRISP

Later in the day you might want to give this little snack a try. Apples and pomegranates are always on hand at my house. If you don't want to peel pomegranates to gather the arils (seeds), you can often buy the arils in plastic tubs.

1/2 cup old-fashioned oats

1/2 cup all-purpose flour

1/2 cup packed brown sugar

  Cinnamon

1/2 stick (4 tablespoons) softened butter

  3 apples, peeled and cored

1/3 cup pomegranate arils

Preheat the oven to 350°F. Combine oats, flour, brown sugar, cinnamon to taste, and butter in a mixing bowl, and mix until the butter is blended well. Chop the apples into bite-size pieces, and spread them out in a baking dish. Add half of the pomegranate arils on top of the apples, then sprinkle the oat mixture and remaining arils on top. Bake for 30 to 35 minutes. Allow to cool before serving.

MAKES 4 SERVINGS

STRAWBERRY-ORANGE SHAKE

I try to keep fresh fruit in the house, but I always have plenty of frozen fruit in my freezer for this quick drink. This low-cal shake is one of my favorite afternoon snacks, so I keep an ice-cube tray of frozen orange juice in my freezer, too. (Note: 1 tray of frozen juice will make about 8 drinks; this recipe makes four drinks, but I often alter it to make just two drinks by halving the remaining ingredients).

2 cups fresh orange juice

8 ounces frozen whole strawberries

1 cup chilled skim milk, rice milk, or soy milk

1/2 cup chilled nonfat plain or vanilla yogurt

Pour the orange juice into an ice-cube tray and freeze until hard, 4 hours or overnight.

Put the frozen strawberries in a blender and add half of the orange juice ice cubes (keep the remaining cubes in the freezer for future use), the milk, and the yogurt. Blend until smooth. Pour into 4 tall glasses and serve with straws.

MAKES ABOUT 4 DRINKS

BECOMING ACCOUNTABLE

I recently joined a new gym right down the street from my apartment. It's within walking distance—just 0.04 miles away—which basically prevents me from making excuses not to go. As part of my new membership, I received a free training session with the owner. I was excited to jump-start my fitness routine, so I scheduled an appointment right away.

At our training session on Tuesday morning, Tom asks me a bunch of standard questions about my health: Do you have any injuries? Do you have any medical conditions that I should know about? What are your goals? He's sort of rambling them off, and

I am responding appropriately as I walk on the treadmill to warm up. Tom seems like he wants to get right to the workout, so he skips a few questions, which is fine with me. I'm ready to get down to business, too. Then he casually asks me about my height and weight for his records. I tell him that I am five feet four inches tall, but I'm not really sure how much I weigh. Tom looks surprised but then asks for a weight range. I tell him 128 to 132 pounds (the last time I checked).

The Unhappy Numbers Game

I don't weigh myself anymore. I used to have a scale and hop on every single day to see where my weight fell. If I had gained even a couple of pounds, the number staring back at me ruined my whole day. I recently threw out my scale because the unhappiness it caused outweighed (no pun intended!) its usefulness.

So, how did I get to this place where I didn't care about numbers any more?

Life was good. Mal and I had just moved into a new apartment—a funky modern loft in South Boston—and I had finally gotten my perfect pug puppy, which I had wanted for years. My blog was starting to take off, and freelance jobs and opportunities were popping up all over the place. Despite my nice little life, I noticed that a few pounds started to creep on. At the time, I was working full-time as the executive assistant to the dean of Harvard College, blogging at *Carrots 'N' Cake*, and doing freelance work for *Health* magazine, so my free time was very limited. Soon, I began skipping my daily gym sessions and opting for convenience over nutrition when it came to food. It really wasn't a surprise that I had gained five pounds from this new lifestyle.

As soon as I noticed that my jeans were a bit tighter than usual, I obsessively weighed myself every day. My morning ritual involved a sweat session followed by a daily weigh and a shower before breakfast. I did this every morning for two weeks—and every day the scale determined how my day would go. I knew that my weight would fluctuate a few pounds because of water weight and other bodily changes, but those little pounds made me crazy. If the number on the scale was down a few pounds, the rest of my day went well. If it was up even just a pound, it instantly put me in a bad mood for the rest of the day.

What Would My Readers Think?

At the same time, I was blogging about healthy living at *Carrots 'N' Cake*. No one knew that I was struggling with the scale. When my weight was within my "feel-great-weight" range, I didn't obsessively check the scale, but now that I had gained a few pounds, I couldn't help myself. What would my readers think? I was the gal who found her "happy" weight through healthy moderation, but here I was standing on the scale every single morning, hoping that the number would make me happy.

I didn't tell my readers about this struggle because I didn't want to let them down. I think many of them look to me as a healthy role model, not someone obsessed with calories and the scale. If I told them that the number on the scale stressed me out, they'd think I was a hypocrite or just a phony.

Eventually, I realized that a lot of people who have lost weight have struggled with maintaining it and that perhaps my readers would rally around me and become a great support system for me. I didn't need to look perfect all of the time. I think a lot of my readers identify with me because I'm so relatable and experience the same types of things they experience. Perhaps my battle with the scale would resonate with them. Plus, I wanted to be open and honest with my readers. They come to *Carrots 'N' Cake* for motivation, advice, and inspiration, so I wanted to make sure that what I was portraying was completely authentic and honest.

As I thought about my blog readers, it soon became clear to me that this whole scale ritual was crazy. A number was determining how I felt about myself, and I knew better than that! How could I blog about living well but obsess over something like a bathroom scale? I felt like a hypocrite and vowed to give up my scale habit forever.

While organizing and cleaning the new apartment, I realized that there was no room for my scale in the bathroom. There was minimal storage under the sink and no closet. Of course, I could have stored my bathroom scale somewhere else in the apartment, but I sort of saw this situation as a sign. Perhaps there was no room for the scale in my life as well. There were boxes and packing materials that needed to be thrown out, so I took my scale and put it on the discard pile. The next morning, when Mal and I were dragging all the trash to the curb, he noticed the scale and asked me if it was supposed to be there. My response: "Oh yeah, that can go."

Now I see that number on the scale as just another number to keep track of in the grand scheme of living a healthy lifestyle. I can't let the number go too high or too low, and I found that I am my happiest within a five-pound weight range. I'm not saying that I never weigh myself—I do—but I only do so every few months at the gym. What's more important to me is knowing what I put into my body.

Misguided Youth

This is going to sound terrible, but I typically ate only two meals a day in college (lunch and dinner), and that, coupled with daily workouts, made it easy for me to maintain my weight, despite drinking a lot of beer and indulging in the occasional cereal binge.

At college, I'd sleep through breakfast and go to my first class of the day around ten thirty. When class was over, I'd eat lunch in the dining hall, usually a ham and cheese sandwich or big salad from the salad bar with chicken breast on top. I'd eat the same thing for dinner. The only snack I'd eat between lunch and dinner was coffee or frozen yogurt. I had some seriously unhealthy habits in college!

I gained about twenty-five pounds after college. I went from a relatively healthy and active lifestyle as an undergraduate to a lazy, beer-drinking twenty-something who sat behind a desk for forty hours per week working at a marketing and promotions company. The majority of my colleagues also were in their twenties, which meant that happy hour and late nights out in the city were the main social scene.

I was going out for beers and bar food at least three nights a week with co-workers. For the most part, my breakfast and lunch were nutritious, but midmorning and afternoon coffee runs with co-workers soon became a common occurrence. A small coffee soon turned into a small coffee and a donut . . . twice a day. Add in nightly plates of nachos, and it wasn't a surprise that I gained so much weight in just a few months.

With a steady diet of pepperoni pizza and giant chocolate chip muffins, instead of salmon-topped salads and Greek yogurt, it wasn't a mystery why I needed to buy a whole new wardrobe (true story!). I thought I could hide from the effects of my new lifestyle, but I needed to be honest with myself—if not for my waistline, then definitely for my health.

Jump Start

I resigned from the job a few months later, but the weight gain was only a symptom of the reasons why. The job was very stressful at times, the hours were long, and the accompanying lifestyle was not good for my health. I took a job working in college admissions at a local university, where the pace was slower and the hours much more reasonable. Taking on a new job was the jump start I needed to get back on track. It was like turning over a new leaf. I wanted to be healthy again.

Leaving my high-stress marketing job meant a considerable pay cut. I enjoyed my new position, but living in Boston, it was difficult to pay all of the bills. So, I decided to get a part-time job at a local health club to supplement my income. One of the perks of working at the front desk, checking people in, was that I could use the facility and take classes for free. My new gig fit right into my new health goals. I started to exercise most mornings of the week before my full-time job. I took Body Pump classes twice a week as well as spinning and step aerobic classes. The club had so many nice amenities, it motivated me to go almost every morning.

I mostly had the fitness element of a healthy lifestyle all figured out, but my eating habits needed some work. At this point, I finally started to take responsibility for what I put into my body. I started tracking what I ate every day using an online calorie counter. For the most part, I was religious about recording my calories for the day, which helped keep me on track.

In college and after college, I really started to see fitness as something important to living a healthy life. In high school, I played team sports—soccer, basketball, tennis, and track—so I almost always had a practice, game, match, or meet to attend. I exercised because it made me better at the sport I played. Plus, my teammates relied on me to play well.

When I got to college, I didn't play team sports, but my friends were really into exercise, especially running and group exercise classes at the gym, which made consistently working out so much easier. I mean, if my friend was going to the gym or for a three-mile run, so should I. It was fun exercising with friends, and it made sticking to it a piece of cake.

After college, however, it was a lot more difficult to exercise. The gym was no longer a quick walk from my apartment, and I didn't have a whole slew of friends living nearby to motivate me to go to the gym. I was on my own, and I finally made a real commitment to fitness.

Of course, every day wasn't perfect. There would be days that I ate seven cookies instead of eating a healthy snack in the afternoon, but that was something I chose to be honest with myself about. Not recording the cookies in my online calorie tracker didn't mean that I didn't eat them. I just needed to step up and accept the responsibility.

I counted calories and tracked calories for years—mostly because it wasn't easy for me to change my eating habits. Tracking calories laid everything out for me: how many calories I was eating and at which meals. It even let me see if I was overdoing unhealthy fats. Looking back on weeks, even months, showed me where I needed to cut calories and fat and where I needed to add protein and fiber.

Real Food

Eventually, I stopped focusing so much on actual calories and started eating "real" food—basically, a lot less of the processed stuff. I found that many of the "diet" foods that I was eating—rice cakes, fiber bars, and nonfat cookies (think Snackwells)—did nothing for my hunger and left me wanting more food later. I found myself always hungry and always craving something more. When I started to fill my diet with more wholesome foods, many of these cravings went away. Plus, I didn't want to consume lots of hard-to-pronounce ingredients, which were often found in the diet products I had been previously eating.

I used FitDay.com to track my calories. It's a free website with a pretty large database of foods to choose from. It also provides an option to add your own foods and save them into the system, which made tracking my calories even easier. It would take me just a few seconds to track each meal. I used FitDay.com for years.

The biggest shocker for me was realizing that I didn't eat nearly enough fresh produce. There were even some days that I didn't eat a single vegetable! I was staying within my calorie-range goal each day, but I wasn't eating wholesome foods. It almost felt like I was cheating because what I was eating included so many low-calorie diet foods. Of course, the number of calories I was consuming was very important to me, but soon I realized that if I wanted to truly be healthy and maintain this lifestyle, I needed to step it up in the nutrition department.

My caloric goal was (and still is) 1,800 to 2,200 calories per day. The only diet that I followed was the "make changes for life diet." After realizing that I couldn't eat diet food forever—it didn't make me happy—I vowed to eat and exercise the right way. I started to read a ton of health and fitness magazines to learn what I should be eating. I knew that if I wanted to lose weight once and for all, I needed to make changes that I could incorporate into my life for good—not just to lose weight. Otherwise, any weight I lost would come right back once I went back to my old ways. It was easy making these changes because I already had a number of ingrained habits, but over time, I found ways to fit in new healthy habits that worked with my current ones.

Nutrition Revisited

Soon, I became almost obsessed with learning more about nutrition. I started reading as many books and magazines as I could get my hands on and spent hours scouring the

Internet. I probably read more books during this time than I did in a whole year of college! I even seriously considered going back to school to become a registered dietitian. The more I learned about nutrition, the easier it became for me to make healthy choices in my diet. I started reading package labels and eliminating as many chemicals (like Splenda) as possible from my diet.

I used an at-home study course from the American Fitness Professionals Association, which took just three months to complete, and became certified as a nutrition and wellness consultant. I learned a ton from the course, and it was great to build that type of nutrition knowledge, especially for my blog.

And learning how to select more nutritious foods actually had a surprising benefit for my appetite: I could eat more! As an afternoon snack, for instance, I plowed through a high-fiber bar so fast that it almost seemed like I didn't eat it. But then I learned that I could enjoy an apple with some peanut butter for about the same amount of calories—and the apple would be much more satisfying both physically and mentally. It would take me longer to eat the apple, and the natural fiber and healthy fats from the peanut butter would keep me satisfied for much longer than the artificial ingredients in the fiber bar.

Once I started making more informed decisions about what I put into my body, I finally felt like I had control over my weight. Even though I never blamed anyone for my original weight gain, I now took responsibility for what my body looked like and how I felt on the inside. And how I felt was no surprise. My outlook on life changed, I started setting goals for myself, and eventually, this feeling of accountability and control led me to want to share my experience with other people.

Healthy Tips: I look for low-calorie ways to boost the flavor in my favorite dishes by keeping a variety of spices right near my stove. I normally reach for garlic powder, ground ginger, cumin, and sea salt. Also, I keep measuring cups and spoons right by my prep area. I used to try to eyeball high-calorie ingredients like oils, butter, and margarine, just like chefs do on cooking shows, but I noticed that I was being too generous with my estimates and it was adding up—1 tablespoon of olive oil, for instance, has 120 calories!

LEMON CHICKEN SKEWERS

Chicken cooked on skewers is fun to eat, and preparing it like this is a good way to limit the amount of protein on my plate. These are delicious and super quick.

2 chicken cutlets

1/4 preserved lemon (store-bought), flesh discarded, peel finely chopped

1 tablespoon olive oil

1 garlic clove, crushed through a press

1/4 teaspoon red pepper flakes, or to taste

1/4 teaspoon dried oregano, crushed

1/4 teaspoon salt

1/4 teaspoon freshly ground black pepper, or to taste

Soak 8 (6-inch) bamboo skewers in water for 30 minutes.

Place the cutlets between sheets of waxed paper on a cutting board, and pound with a rolling pin or meat mallet until ¼-inch thick. Cut the pieces into 1-inch-wide strips.

Combine the preserved lemon, oil, garlic, pepper flakes, oregano, salt, and pepper in a bowl, and mix well. Add the chicken and toss to coat.

Preheat the broiler. Line a baking sheet with foil. Thread the chicken strips onto the skewers. Place the skewers on the prepared baking sheet and broil the chicken about 6 inches from the heat source until cooked through, 1 to 2 minutes.

MAKES 8 SMALL SKEWERS

3-MINUTE OATMEAL RAISIN COOKIE

Need to stave off a sudden craving? Here's a giant cookie that takes just minutes to make.

- 1/4 cup oats
- 1/8 cup liquid egg whites
- 2 teaspoons brown sugar
- 2 teaspoons all-purpose flour
- 1/4 teaspoon vanilla extract
- 1/4 teaspoon baking powder
- 1 tablespoon raisins
-    Cinnamon to taste

Combine all ingredients in a microwave-safe bowl. Scrape batter down the sides of the bowl and flatten into a cookie shape at the bottom. Place the bowl in the microwave and cook for 45 seconds on high.

Allow to cool, remove the cookie from the bowl, and enjoy!

MAKES 1 GIANT COOKIE

BLUEBERRY BRAN MUFFINS

Packed with bran and blueberries, these muffins make a good alter-native to lots of other goodies. They always satisfy my sweet tooth.

1 cup unprocessed oat bran

1 cup all-purpose flour

1/2 cup stone-ground whole wheat flour

11/4 teaspoons baking powder

1 teaspoon ground cinnamon

1/2 teaspoon baking soda

1/2 teaspoon salt

1/3 cup honey

1/4 cup canola oil

1 egg

11/4 cups buttermilk

1 cup fresh or frozen blueberries

Preheat the oven to 400°F and grease 12 muffin cups with nonstick cooking spray.

Combine the bran, flours, baking powder, cinnamon, baking soda, and salt in a large bowl. Whisk the honey, oil, and egg in a small bowl just until blended. Whisk in the butter-milk, and pour into the bran mixture. Whisk just until the dry ingredients are moistened. Stir in the blueberries, and spoon the batter into the prepared muffin cups.

Bake the muffins until a cake tester inserted in the center comes out clean, about 20 minutes. Remove the muffins from the pans, and cool briefly on a wire rack.

MAKES 12 MUFFINS

MAINTAINING MY WEIGHT: WHAT WORKS

Nowadays, after another Saturday night with a heavy meal out and one too many glasses of wine, I'm once again looking to get myself back on track. I'm fine with getting a little off track every now and then. I want to enjoy life, and sometimes I do that through food and drink. I'd rather be happy than miserable because of a diet that restricts me from my favorite foods. I just have to make sure I indulge within reason.

Looking back on the weekend, I realize that I enjoyed a lot of carbs. Don't get me wrong—I love carbs, but I definitely loaded up on the not-so-good kind. On Sunday morning, I vowed to eat a healthy yet light breakfast and lunch, filled with whole grains and fruit, followed by a big salad for dinner. I knew some whole grains and fresh produce would make me feel better after such an unhealthy weekend of eating.

My Blog Buddies and Me

A few months ago, I attended a food-blogger festival in San Francisco. It was a great time to meet up with some of my online friends in person and explore the city. Of course, I enjoyed eating and drinking my little heart out!

This was quite the special occasion—San Francisco with my blog buddies to attend a food festival. The whole point was to eat, drink, and be merry, so I embraced it. I let myself get a little crazy and enjoyed myself, but I made sure to incorporate some light meals and exercise to help balance out all of the splurges. It was such an amazing opportunity; I didn't want to spend it stressing out about calories and fat. Some of us joked that on our indulgent weekend, no carb was left behind. Of course, we thought this little saying was pretty funny, but the more I thought about it, the more I realized that though the Atkins rage ended years ago, carbs still get a bad rap—even among my healthy, foodie friends.

Carb Crazy

Before I lost more than twenty pounds, I tried all kinds of low-carb diets—most notably the Atkins Diet. I would load my grocery cart with meat, cheese, and eggs and avoid oatmeal and brightly colored fruits like the plague. In the month that I devoted myself to Atkins, I ate eggs almost

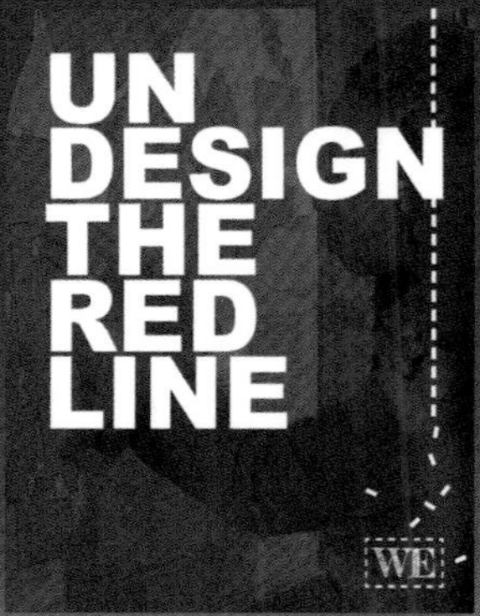

Handwritten annotations:

www.hclibrary.org

TOURS {
  Sat. @ 11am.
  Tues @ 7pm.
  Thurs @ 1pm.
}

UN DESIGN THE RED LINE

WE

Untangle the roots of housing discrimination

THROUGH DECEMBER 31

Howard County Library System
Central Branch (10375 Little Patuxent Pkwy, Columbia)

hclibrary.org

This interactive exhibit explores the history of structural racism and classism, how these designs compounded each other from redlining maps until today, and how we can come together to undesign these systems intentionally.

Sponsored by Columbia Association, Enterprise Community Partners, Friends & Foundation of HCLS, Howard Community College, #OneHoward, and the Institute of Museum and Library Services.

View by yourself or with a group. Call 410.313.7800 or visit **choosecivility.org** to sign up for a guided tour.

Email redline@hclibrary.org to schedule a group tour.

Visit **choosecivility.org** for a list of related events, readings, and resources.

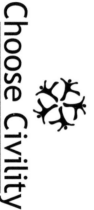

Choose Civility
HOWARD COUNTY, MD

every day for breakfast. I even ate an entire block of cheese more than once. And the whole time that I was on the Atkins Diet, I felt cranky and lethargic. I was not pleasant to be around—my poor roommate at the time must have wanted to kill me! Of course, I questioned how healthy this diet could really be—especially since I hadn't eaten a piece of fruit in weeks—but the pounds soon came off, and that motivated me to stick with it.

As with most restrictive diets, I eventually caved in and binged on carbs, especially the unhealthy kind, like doughnuts, enormous chocolate chip muffins, and nachos. Eating those types of foods didn't make me feel much better, but it did make me realize that I needed carbs in my diet— the good kind, of course—in order to function. So after my brief stint with Atkins, I vowed to incorporate healthy carbs back into my diet, and as soon as I did, my mood and energy levels improved almost instantly. The key was finally figuring out the right kinds of carbs to eat. Sure, I knew that a candy bar provided a different type of carb than steamed broccoli, but how did my morning bagel fit into that equation? If the bag said whole wheat, could I consider it a good carb? I was definitely carb confused. It took me a while to banish Atkins- and South Beach–inspired rules from my mind. I don't like to categorize foods as "good" and "bad," but it's no secret that complex carbs satisfy me longer and I don't feel that blood-sugar crash.

The Truth About Salads

While losing weight, I learned which foods satisfy me and which do not. One of the biggest surprises for a seemingly diet-friendly food was salad. Everyone who goes on a diet—including me!—thinks that salads are automatically a safe diet food. Salads are a great way to pack more veggies into your diet, but the calories can also start to show up on the scale if you aren't careful. Over the years, I learned how to eat a more nutritious, low-calorie salad.

The Three-quarters Rule

The most helpful rule that I created for myself is what I call the "three-quarters rule." I used to make a number of simple mistakes at the salad bar. I thought I was creating healthy salads, but I was loading up on high-calorie ingredients. I chose full-fat cheeses, iceberg lettuce, and starchy carbohydrates like pasta salad and croutons. I thought that as long as they were served over greens, they were healthy. Boy, was I wrong! At the same time, I avoided high-calorie healthy fats like nuts, olives, and avocados, but now I realize that these healthy fats are good for me and help me feel full for hours. So when making a salad, I apply the three-quarters rule. Three-quarters of my salad is made up of leafy greens and raw veggies, while one-quarter is devoted to small portions of healthy fats and higher-calorie "fun" ingredients. That way, my salads never get boring, and I never feel like I'm depriving myself.

Dressing on the Side, Please

When dining out, I always thought that asking for my salad dressing on the side was the healthy, low-calorie option. But, now I think twice about doing this because I realize that I was dipping every piece of my salad into the dressing and eating the entire portion anyway. I still ask for my salad dressing on the side, but I pour a small amount onto my salad and lightly dress it myself. This way, I avoid a salad drenched in dressing, but I don't feel deprived or miss the flavor. My favorite dressings are actually very simple: a sprinkle of balsamic vinegar and olive oil, or a homemade mix of chopped cucumber, low-fat plain yogurt, fresh dill, and lemon juice.

I used to make the same salad day after day, which, as you can imagine, ended up being boring and unappetizing. Now I don't let myself get into a salad rut; instead, I experiment with interesting ingredients and try to think outside the box when preparing my homemade salads. Perusing the farmers' market, for example, always gives me ideas. Recently, I've been experimenting with fresh herbs—particularly basil and dill. The natural flavors are lightly present throughout my entire salad, so I often don't need to add dressing. And while I always try to add some colorful veggies for their nutritional benefits, I like to have fun too. Almost anything goes! My favorite ingredients include pecans, chickpeas, sprouts, kiwi slices, goat cheese, pumpkin seeds, and even falafel, but I'm always looking for new additions to keep things interesting.

ZUCCHINI AND CHICKPEA SALAD

The beauty of this little salad is that I usually have all the ingredients on hand, so I can whip it up without having to run out to the store. It's just right for a light lunch or a healthy snack.

1 medium zucchini, finely chopped

1 large yellow bell pepper, diced

1/2 cup sliced radishes

1 (15-ounce) can chickpeas, drained and rinsed

1/3 cup no-salt-added tomato juice

1/4 cup olive oil

1/4 cup red wine vinegar

1/2 teaspoon freshly ground black pepper

1/2 teaspoon dried oregano, crushed

1/2 teaspoon dry mustard

1/4 teaspoon light soy sauce

1/8 teaspoon cayenne

Combine zucchini, bell pepper, radishes, and chickpeas in a large bowl, and toss to mix. Put the remaining ingredients in a jar, seal with a tight-fitting lid, and shake vigorously until mixed thoroughly. Drizzle some of the tomato vinaigrette over the salad, and toss until vegetables are coated lightly. Store any remaining vinaigrette in the refrigerator.

MAKES 2 SERVINGS

DOUBLE-TOMATO BRUSCHETTA

My favorite Italian restaurant serves bruschetta as a starter, but I often make a batch for lunch with a bowl of soup.

3 sun-dried tomato halves (not in oil)

1/2 cup basil leaves

1/4 cup extra-virgin olive oil

3 ripe plum tomatoes, seeded and diced

3/4 cup diced smoked mozzarella cheese

1 tablespoon red wine vinegar

1/4 teaspoon salt

Four slices rustic Italian bread

Preheat the oven to 350°F.

To make the tomato-basil oil, place the dried tomatoes in a heat-safe bowl and add ¼ cup boiling water. Let soak for 5 minutes. Drain, pat dry, and mince. Mince half of the basil leaves. Combine the minced basil and tomatoes in a small bowl. Add 2 tablespoons olive oil, and mix well. Set aside.

Stack the remaining basil leaves and thinly slice crosswise into shreds. Place in a medium bowl, and add the remaining 2 tablespoons olive oil, the fresh tomatoes, cheese, vinegar, and salt. Mix well.

Brush the bread slices on both sides with the tomato-basil oil. Arrange the bread on a baking sheet, and bake until golden and crisp, 8 to 10 minutes. Top with the fresh tomato mixture, and serve immediately.

MAKES 4 BRUSCHETTA

SPINACH-TOMATO
EGG WHITE OMELET

Whenever I want to watch what I eat and still feel pampered, I make this omelet—sometimes for lunch and sometimes for dinner.

4 egg whites

1 tablespoon water

1/8 teaspoon kosher salt

1/8 teaspoon freshly ground black pepper

1 teaspoon olive oil

2 tablespoons shredded reduced-fat cheddar cheese

1/2 cup shredded spinach leaves

1/4 cup chopped tomato

Combine the egg whites, water, salt, and pepper in a bowl, and whisk to combine.

Heat the oil in an 8-inch nonstick skillet over medium-high heat, and add the eggwhite mixture. Tilt the pan to spread the mixture over the bottom, and cook until set, 1 to 2 minutes, using a heat-safe plastic spatula to constantly lift the edges of the egg to allow the uncooked portion to flow underneath. Sprinkle with the cheese, spinach leaves, and tomato, and slide onto a plate, folding the omelet over by lifting the handle of the skillet as the omelet comes out.

MAKES 1 SERVING

FRESH FRUIT SALAD

Fruit should be part of everyone's daily diet, and this salad combines all my favorites. The dressing is so good, you'll want to put it on everything. As for the nutmeg, it will make a world of difference if you grate your own. You can find whole nutmeg in the grocery store; simply grate it using the smallest holes of your grater.

2 mangoes, pitted, peeled, and cut into chunks

1 orange, peeled and cut into sections

1 banana, peeled and cut crosswise into 1/4-inch rounds

1 kiwi, peeled, quartered lengthwise, and cut crosswise
    into 1/2-inch-thick chunks

1 cup fresh grapefruit sections

1 cup ripe cantaloupe chunks

1 cup low-fat vanilla yogurt

2 tablespoons fresh lime juice

1/8 teaspoon grated nutmeg, or more to taste

1/2 teaspoon coarsely ground black pepper

1/4 teaspoon salt

Combine the fruit in a nonreactive bowl, and mix gently. Put the yogurt, lime juice, nutmeg, pepper, and salt in a blender, and blend until smooth. Drizzle dressing over fruit, and toss to coat.

MAKES 4 SERVINGS FOR DESSERT

7

PAYING ATTENTION

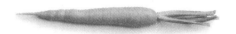

Today I met my sister Steph after work for holiday shopping and then dinner. Hanging out with her is always a fun time. She's my only sibling and just fifteen months younger than me, so she's basically my best friend. We live only about thirty minutes away from each other, so we're together quite often after work and on the weekends.

Spending time with my sister is also easy and stress free because we are so much alike. I'm definitely a more type A personality than she, but for the most part we both go with the flow. We have the same goofy sense of humor that we share with our husbands, so when the four of us get together, there's a lot of laughter. Steph and I actually got married at the exact same age—she married almost exactly fifteen months after me. She works in higher education, just like I did for so many years, and we love many of the same things, like cooking, fitness, animals, shopping, and a good beer.

Making Choices

Steph and I decide where to shop and where to eat dinner in about ten seconds. We decide to visit the Christmas Tree Shop for affordable holiday decorations and stocking stuffers, and then we hit up Kohl's for a gift for my mother. Dinner is an easy choice too: Pizzeria Regina. It's one of our favorite pizza places, and it's nearby, so just like that our evening is planned.

At the Christmas Tree Shop, we have a little trouble focusing at first. We start off wandering the store and getting distracted by sales and holiday deals. We even begin shopping for ourselves, which is the exact opposite of why we're out together. Eventually, we pull out our shopping list and focus on the task at hand. We find all sorts of stocking stuffers and a few holiday decorations for each of our homes. After about an hour, we're at the cash register. Then we head to Kohl's, which is a totally different experience. We know exactly what we want to get my mom for Christmas. We came prepared. We even have a store coupon. We're in and out of the store in record time and heading straight to dinner.

When we arrive at Pizzeria Regina, I am famished. I missed my usual afternoon snack today, so it's been a good seven hours since I have eaten anything. My sister is hungry too, so as soon as we sit down at the table, we order a large vegetable pizza to share. Gotta get those veggies in where I can!

While we wait for our order, we chat about our recent purchases and what our plans are for Christmas. We split our time between Mom and Dad, both sets of grandparents, and our in-laws, so the day definitely takes some serious coordination. By the time we've come up with a tentative Christmas Day game plan, our pizza arrives and our conversation abruptly ends. It's time to eat!

"I Win"

We practically barrel through a slice each before taking a second to breathe. My sister finishes her piece before me. "I win," she jokes, as if we were in an eating competition. I laugh, but realize I barely even tasted my food because I was eating so fast. I didn't really enjoy it at all. When I'm famished, it's so easy to eat mindlessly without paying attention to the I help myself to a second slice of pizza but make a conscious effort to eat this one more slowly. I decide to eat this slice with a fork and a knife, which slows my pace and helps me to savor each bite and really enjoy the experience. I pause between bites and chew each one completely. I taste all the flavors—the bell peppers, onions, garlic, and even black olives, which I missed while eating the first slice.

I tell Steph that the second slice of pizza tasted so much better than the first. She's slowed her eating pace too and agrees. We both debate whether to have a third piece, but eating the second piece so slowly allowed our bodies to register that we'd had enough to eat. We ask for the rest of the pizza to be split into two boxes so we can both take some home for leftovers.

My sister's innocent statement, "I win," got me thinking about paying attention to how and what I eat—not just in terms of calories or healthy versus not healthy, but in terms of flavor. In general, I'm pretty good at pacing myself. If I cook dinner at home, I have no problem giving the meal that I am eating some extra attention. Mostly likely, I have cooked it from scratch, so I appreciate the process and don't want to wolf it down. I've just spent an hour cooking, so I want to enjoy the results. Sometimes, though, it can be tough—like when I haven't eaten for seven hours and a big cheesy pizza is placed right in front of me! I hate feeling hungry, so it's a toss-up whether I gorge or savor.

Typically, I eat three meals with one or two snacks thrown into the mix. Most days, I'll eat a small snack between breakfast and lunch and then another between lunch and dinner. These snacks are usually about 200 calories each and consist of high-fiber carbs mixed with a bit of protein and fat, like half of a whole-wheat English muffin with peanut butter spread on top.

Focus and Enjoy

Over time, I've learned to make eating a special occasion, especially at a restaurant, where I pay someone to make a beautiful meal for me to enjoy. I don't have to do a thing except eat, so why wouldn't I think of it as an event? I also respect the food that someone has made for me, so I make sure to focus on the experience and enjoy every second.

When I dine out, I like to enjoy myself. I don't want

to stress about what to order, and I don't need to know what the "healthiest" option is on the menu or how a dish is prepared. While I do ask for my salad dressing on the side, I don't get caught up in the whole "twenty questions about what's in it and how it's cooked" thing. Having someone make a nice meal and serve it to me is a special experience. I enjoy every part of it.

Think Small

That doesn't mean I don't think about what I'm going to eat. I always take a couple of minutes to peruse the menu. My eyes always focus on the same menu headings: salads, soups, sandwiches, appetizers, side dishes, and specials. I find that these menu categories offer the healthiest dining-out options—often in smaller portions than the main courses. I like to indulge a little when I eat out, but portion size is key to keeping my calories and fat in check for the day.

It seems like you actually have to go out of your way to get a small size when you dine or order out. Ordering a large salad for dinner is one thing, but how about the large latte or large French fries? They're not healthy options. Plus, eateries give you a financial incentive of sorts to order the large size. You can "supersize" your meal for just a dollar. Who wouldn't want to take advantage of that deal?

There's nothing wrong with ordering a small portion. Most of the time, I eat it and feel completely satisfied. If I order a regular-size meal, chances are that I'll get just as full without eating the whole thing: I can always stop and reassess if I want to eat more. I usually find that the small size is just right. Plus, I love being able to sample lots of different foods, so ordering a bunch of small plates allows me to satisfy all of my cravings without eating too many calories.

At home, I try to make my food as special as possible, so I am more likely to pay attention to what I eat and make meals and snacks an experience. Consider a homemade salad. I can easily cut up some lettuce, tomatoes, and cucumbers, add some dressing, and call it a salad. But why not make that salad something special? I like to add fresh goat cheese, grilled sweet potato, pumpkin seeds, tiny gherkins, and other ingredients that will upgrade my salad and make it worth taking the time to enjoy. I'll season my salad with ground pepper, fresh basil, even dried rosemary—and a little balsamic vinegar and olive oil go a long way toward jazzing up the flavor of any salad. Taking a little extra time to make my meal special helps me to be much more satisfied with my food. It also helps me savor each bite and make the process of preparing and eating food that much more special.

My Tips for Slowing Down When Eating

I make it special. More than once, I've stood in my kitchen and chowed down a snack that I just prepared. But keeping my weight loss in mind, I now put in the effort to make my meals and snacks a little more special. For example, instead of just peeling a banana and eating it as is, I slice it, put it in an attractive bowl, and top it with chopped walnuts and honey. Increasing the specialness of my snack makes me appreciate it more and really savor it.

I pause before my first bite. Before I even taste my

food, I take a moment to relax and consider my hunger level. This reminds me to slow down, which ultimately leads me to consume fewer calories. Plus, making it a point to pause before my meal allows me to focus on the meal and really enjoy it.

I put down my fork. It usually takes me about 20 minutes to feel satisfied while eating a meal, so I find it helpful to put down my fork after every few bites to stay in tune with my body's fullness. Keeping tabs on my satisfaction throughout my meal helps me eat slower.

Most people losing weight would likely put fast food on their forbidden list, but in a pinch it's sometimes my only option. Plus, my husband loves the stuff—particularly a sausage, egg, and cheese on a plain bagel from Dunkin' Donuts—so sometimes I just can't avoid it.

I try to eat mostly healthy when it comes to fast food, so I commend these places for at least trying to incorporate healthier options. McDonald's has sliced apples and Burger King has veggie burgers, which are better than French fries and Whoppers if you must eat fast food. However, I don't see these "healthier" options as an excuse to eat fast food over real food. Having healthy menu options available isn't going to keep my weight steady if I eat fast food all the time. Basically, there is no quick fix for weight loss, and I keep this in mind every time I splurge on fast food.

While I don't eat fast food all that often, I have to admit to occasionally ordering a turkey bacon and egg sandwich from Starbucks or a skinny latte from Dunkin' Donuts when I'm in a rush. But I make sure to stick to a few rules when I do:

My Tips for Eating Fast Food

I drink water with my meal. If I'm going to indulge in fast food, I skip the soda altogether. Even if you order a zero-calorie diet soda, there is nothing nutritious about it!

I always order small. This obviously helps reduce unneeded calories and fat. If the "small" isn't actually that small, I'll share it with my husband or take the other half home for later.

I nix the extras. For example, if I order a mocha from Starbucks, I don't need to have whipped cream too.

I enjoy the splurge—and don't feel guilty about it! Of course, moderation is key, but if I overdo it, I just get back on track the next day with extra-healthy meals and some exercise.

BROWN SUGAR–BALSAMIC DATE PIZZA WITH CARAMELIZED ONIONS, WALNUTS, AND FETA

There are so many wonderful, bold flavors in this pizza. The caramelized onions and feta combined with the brown sugar and balsamic vinegar give it an instant flavor boost.

1/2 tablespoon olive oil

1 tablespoon chopped white onion

5 pitted dates, chopped into 1/4-inch pieces

1/2 tablespoon brown sugar

1 tablespoon balsamic vinegar

1 whole wheat pita (leave it whole)

2 teaspoons chopped walnuts

1 tablespoon crumbled feta

Preheat the oven to 350°F. In a small sauté pan, heat the olive oil; then add the onion and dates. Sauté until onions are soft. Meanwhile, in a small bowl, mix the brown sugar with the balsamic vinegar.

Drizzle the balsamic vinegar–brown sugar mixture on top of the pita, then top with onion, dates, walnuts, and feta.

Cook your pita pizza in the oven for 8 to 10 minutes, until the feta melts and the edges of the crust start to brown.

MAKES 1 PITA PIZZA

EASY EGGPLANT PIZZA

Here's another easy pizza that I often throw together with store-bought dough and caponata. I try to limit myself to two pieces, though that doesn't always happen.

---

1 small green zucchini, trimmed and shredded on the
  diagonal

1 small yellow zucchini, trimmed and shredded on the
  diagonal

1 teaspoon salt

  Cornmeal for sprinkling

12 ounces store-bought pizza dough

3/4 cup store-bought caponata

1 cup (4 ounces) shredded mozzarella cheese

Preheat the oven to 450°F. Put the green and yellow zucchini in a bowl, sprinkle with the salt, and toss to coat. Let the mixture stand at least 10 minutes to sweat the vegetables.

Meanwhile, spray a 12-inch pizza pan with nonstick cooking spray and sprinkle with cornmeal. On a floured surface, roll out the pizza dough to a 13-inch round. Transfer the dough to the pan, fold the edge in about ½ inch, and crimp.

Rinse the salt off the zucchini and pat dry with paper towels. Spread the caponata evenly on the dough. Sprinkle evenly with the zucchini and then the mozzarella.

Bake the pizza until crisp, about 15 minutes.

MAKES 1 (12-INCH) PIZZA

TURKEY BURGERS
WITH GRILLED TOMATOES

Everyone loves a big beefy burger now and then, but you can save a zillion calories by making turkey burgers instead and serving them without buns. These burgers have a bit of turkey sausage for added flavor. Even so, each one is only 200 calories!

---

1 pound lean ground turkey

1/2 pound lean turkey sausage, casing removed
       and crumbled

3 green onions, finely chopped

1 celery rib, finely chopped

1 medium zucchini, finely grated

1 garlic clove, crushed through a press

1 teaspoon dried oregano leaves, crushed

1 teaspoon freshly ground black pepper

2 teaspoons soy sauce

3 ripe tomatoes, cut crosswise into 1/2-inch slices

6 Boston lettuce leaves, washed and dried

Combine the turkey, sausage, green onions, celery, zucchini, garlic, oregano, ½ teaspoon pepper, and soy sauce in a bowl and mix gently. With wet hands, shape into 6 (½-inch-thick) patties.

Preheat the broiler, and place the burgers on an aluminum foil–lined baking sheet. Broil the burgers 4 inches from the heat source until cooked through, 8 to 9 minutes, turning over after 6 minutes. Remove the burgers from the heat (keeping the broiler on), and transfer them from the foil to a platter. Let stand, covered, for 3 minutes.

Meanwhile, put a clean piece of aluminum foil on the baking sheet and place the tomatoes on the sheet. Broil the tomatoes until charred and hot, 5 minutes, turning once and sprinkling with the remaining ½ teaspoon pepper.

Place the lettuce leaves on dinner plates, and top each with a burger. Top each burger with a tomato slice, and serve.

MAKES 6 BURGERS

ZUCCHINI AND MUSHROOM BURGERS

I serve these veggie burgers on whole wheat buns or lettuce leaves, your choice, with all the usual toppings.

1 small zucchini, shredded

1 small yellow squash, shredded

1 tablespoon soy sauce

1 tablespoon olive oil

1/2 cup finely chopped onion

1 garlic clove, crushed through a press

1/2 cup chopped fresh shiitake mushrooms

3/4 cup plain dry bread crumbs

1 teaspoon dried Italian herb seasoning mix

1 egg, slightly beaten

1 cup shredded skim-milk mozzarella cheese (optional)

Combine the zucchini, yellow squash, and soy sauce in a large bowl, and toss to coat. Let stand for 10 minutes; then pour the zucchini mixture into a colander and squeeze out most of the liquid. Blot up the rest with paper towels.

Heat the oil in a large nonstick skillet over medium heat until hot. Sauté the onion and garlic until softened and fragrant, about 4 minutes. Add the mushrooms, and sauté until softened, about 3 minutes. Remove the pan from the heat, and add the zucchini, bread crumbs, seasoning mix, egg, and mozzarella (if using). Stir to mix, and form into 4 patties.

Preheat the broiler. Place the burgers on an aluminum foil–lined baking sheet, and broil, turning once, until browned on both sides and the internal temperature registers 160°F, about 10 minutes.

MAKES 4 BURGERS

CHERRY-COCONUT
BAKED APPLES

Baked apples are a best friend to someone looking for a healthy dessert option. Apples are high in fiber, low in calories, and full of flavor, especially when baked with all these goodies.

4	large apples (I used Macoun, but just about any would work)
1/2	cup dried cherries
1/2	cup shredded coconut
1	teaspoon ground cinnamon
1/2	teaspoon grated nutmeg
1	teaspoon vanilla extract
4	teaspoons butter, softened
1/4	cup bread crumbs
2 to 3	teaspoons agave nectar or honey
1	egg
	Vanilla ice cream or frozen yogurt for serving (optional)

Preheat the oven to 350°F and spray an 8-inch square baking dish with nonstick cooking spray. Core but do not peel the apples, and set them in the baking dish.

In a mixing bowl, combine the cherries, coconut, cinnamon, nutmeg, vanilla, butter, breadcrumbs, agave nectar, and egg. Blend well, and fill the center of each apple with the mixture.

Bake for 35 to 40 minutes, until the apples are tender. Serve warm, with ice cream or frozen yogurt if you like.

MAKES 4 SERVINGS

SAUTÉED PEACHES

Sweet, simple, fast—this is my go-to dessert when bushels of ripe peaches appear at the farmers' market.

1 tablespoon sugar

1 teaspoon ground cinnamon

4 peaches, each pitted and cut into 8 wedges

2 tablespoons water

1 cup low-fat peach yogurt

Stir together sugar and cinnamon in a small cup. Grease a large nonstick skillet with nonstick cooking spray, and heat over medium-high heat. Add the peaches, and sauté until hot, about 3 minutes. Sprinkle the peaches with the cinnamon-sugar, and sauté until golden, about 3 minutes more. Add the water, and cook until heated through and juicy, about 3 minutes more. Serve in dessert dishes with a dollop of yogurt on top.

MAKES 4 SERVINGS

8

CRAVINGS AND THE DREADED BINGE

I wake up extra early today to bake breakfast. Sometimes, my love of baking motivates me to do strange things, like wake up super early when I could easily sleep in. Last night, I had a major craving for pumpkin muffins. I'm actually pretty efficient when it comes to baking, so making a batch of muffins first thing in the morning puts me back only about 20 minutes, which is totally worth it for warm, freshly baked muffins.

After mixing up the batter and putting it in the oven to bake, I go along with my normal morning routine: shower, dress, makeup, coffee, check e-mail. I'm also pretty efficient with my morning routine. From start to finish, I can get everything done in the amount of time that it takes the muffins to bake.

Blind Bliss

When the oven timer goes off, I remove the tray from the oven and wait patiently for the muffins to cool. I'm starving, so it's tough to resist the aroma of cinnamon and pumpkin spice. I decide that I can't wait any longer and grab a hot muffin right out of the muffin tray. It practically burns my hand as I reach for a plate. I break the muffin open with my hands and out comes a huge puff of steam. Immediately, I think: butter. Butter would melt so well on this piping-hot, freshly baked muffin, so I grab it from the refrigerator and start spreading it liberally with a butter knife. Five seconds later, I sink my teeth into the muffin. It's so delicious that any thought of photographing it first for the blog goes right out of my head.

While munching on my first muffin, I prepare a second muffin for its photo shoot. I cut it open with the butter knife like a true foodie—not someone ready to chow down. I grab a small, square, white ceramic plate that will look sharp and clean under the orange-colored muffin and go well with the teal placemats on my kitchen table. I then spread a little pat of butter smoothly and evenly on each side of the muffin and let it melt slightly before I snap away. I make sure to position the plate so it receives as much natural sunlight as possible (daylight is the best option for food photography). I snap four or five photos of the muffin before I get the shot that I want to use on my blog. At this point, the muffin has cooled and the butter is melted to perfection. I can't let this delicious baked good go to waste, so I eat it right up.

The second pumpkin muffin leaves a delicious taste in my mouth long after I take my final bite. In fact, I can't stop thinking about how amazing it tasted. Not even five minutes later, I find myself back in the kitchen ready to spread butter on another right-out-of-the-oven pumpkin muffin. Again, I split it open, spread the butter, and pop both halves in my mouth, one after the other. Before I know it, I grab a fourth muffin and do the exact same thing. My brain doesn't even register that I've eaten three already—in fact, my mouth and my brain are totally disconnected. My taste buds are in charge, and they want warm, freshly baked pumpkin muffins.

Out of Sight, Out of Mind

After finishing the fourth muffin, I come to my senses and leave the kitchen completely. I distract myself by watching TV for a little while, but before I know it, I'm eating a fifth muffin. What is going on here? Five muffins in one sitting? I tell myself that I need to stop. I enjoy the last bite of muffin and pack up the remaining muffins in a big Tupperware container. I put the Tupperware container in one of our kitchen cabinets. Out of sight, out of mind. Then I decide that the best way to distract myself from downing more pumpkin muffins and to offset some of the calories would be some exercise.

When I was a kid, food was always a reward, typically in celebration of something really great that happened in my life or my family's life. For instance, getting a good report card at the end of the year always meant a trip to Kimball Farm for ice cream. I swear, I always worked my hardest in the last month of school!

I suppose I've always associated tasty food with happiness, perhaps even being carefree. So as I got older and had to deal with more stresses in life, I looked to food as a way to bring me happiness and deal with this stress. Eating a cookie or brownie made me happy and helped my mind focus on something other than what was bothering me. Food almost seemed an escape for me. Nothing in my life was that bad if I had a piece of cake by my side.

Get Out and Move

But I've also always enjoyed exercise. I started dance lessons as a three-year-old and soccer around age eight, so physical activity has always been in my life. I danced and played soccer because I enjoyed it. As I got older, I still enjoyed participating in sports. In addition to soccer, I played basketball and tennis and ran track in high school. In my off-season from sports, I kept active by taking step aerobics classes at a local gym. I can't remember specifically taking these classes to maintain my weight. I just wanted to exercise since it made me feel good about myself. I loved the choreography and challenge of learning new moves in the step aerobics classes. I was also pretty good at it! I was the youngest person in the class and probably the most coordinated. I guess I got a high from exercising and being so good at it.

In college, I continued to take step aerobics classes, but they met only twice a week during the semester. I started running as a way to stay active and burn (beer) calories. Plus, running seemed to be the cool thing to do at my college. A lot of my friends ran around campus for exercise, so I did it too. I soon realized that in addition to helping me burn calories and feel good about myself, running was a complete stress reliever for me. If I was stressed out about my course work or a fight that I had with my boyfriend, I could throw on my sneakers and escape from everything for 45 minutes. While I ran, my mind wandered and I was able to think through things, which made me feel like I could better deal with the situation. It also helped me think about what I should do to make the situation better. I felt more relaxed and in control after a run.

When I overeat, it almost always stems from feeling stressed or anxious. Eating is an escape from that tense feeling—at least for a little while. Thinking about how delicious the food tastes prevents me from thinking about other things that stress me out. With the muffins, I must have been feeling some sort of stress. I started out just trying a muffin, which tasted good, and then I couldn't stop myself. Maybe I was feeling stressed because I felt like I had no control around them once I had eaten one. Or maybe it was because I was alone and I could eat as many as I wanted in private. I think the more muffins I ate, the more anxious I felt about the whole situation. Having one or two muffins isn't a big deal, but the more I ate, the more guilty I felt about eating them, and then things just spiraled from there.

One of my favorite comfort foods is sugary cereal and milk. It reminds me of my childhood, and it comes in an almost unlimited portion. I recall a specific incident in college when I made my way, bowlful by bowlful, through an entire box of Honey Bunches of Oats. How did I let that happen? Why couldn't I stop myself? How many calories did I consume? It was not a pretty sight.

I always ate while studying—in high school and in college. I found that I couldn't focus unless I had a bag of candy, a muffin, or at least a cup of coffee in my hand. Even today, I don't like to face the computer screen without a cup of tea for comfort. Eating something seems to sooth my anxiety about working or studying so I can focus on what I need to get accomplished. If I don't have something sweet to snack on, I feel stressed about not doing a good job or failing an exam. Eating something sweet relaxes me and makes my workload seem much more manageable—at least for a little while.

A Few Tricks

Now, most of the time, I stop at two bowls of cereal. I also go into pouring myself a bowl knowing that cereal is a trigger food for me. I always plan to have one bowl, but I consciously "allow" myself to have two. Once I've had two bowls, I immediately put my cereal bowl in the sink and fill it with water. I'm too lazy to clean it and pour myself another bowl, and I don't want to dirty another bowl, so this trick really works for me. But, of course, it wasn't always this easy. I've struggled to find a trick like this that works. There was a lot of trial and error for me to get to this point.

I think a lot of my success came with not being so hard on myself. When I tried something new with my cereal binges and it didn't work, I didn't get down in the dumps and beat myself up for it. I looked back at the experience and figured out how I could improve. Not having cereal at all in the house made it seem like a "bad" food to me. So anytime it was in the house, I'd end up binging on it. I needed to figure out a way to feel in control when there was a box of cereal in the house, which, for me, meant getting in the right frame of mind. The first few times, I basically gave myself a pep talk before even digging into the cereal. I knew I was feeling anxious, so I did everything possible to get myself in control of the situation. Essentially, I gave myself a game plan for eating and enjoying a bowl or two of cereal. The first few times, I struggled with keeping my portion to one or two bowls, but eventually, it stuck. Nowadays, I've come to accept that eating two bowls of cereal is the way to go for me. I enjoy the cereal, relieve some of my stress, and feel satisfied after eating two bowls.

I'm definitely in a different mind-set when a binge occurs. A planned splurge is usually exactly that—planned. I think about it ahead of time, and I am much more in control of the situation. I can sit down and enjoy a dessert and stop myself. It's all mental for me in this way. When a binge happens, I am totally out of control. Usually, I am not prepared for it, so when it happens, it's really tough for me to get in control again. Something takes over, and I can't seem to stop myself. These two instances are different too because I really enjoy the indulgence and I don't enjoy the binge as much, especially in regard to how I feel after the experience.

Overeating is the worst feeling. I feel like I have been defeated—like my cravings have taken over and I am powerless to resist them. I feel weak and disappointed in myself. I try not to let these feelings take over because I know nothing good can come from them. But here I am, blogging about healthy living and trying to set a good example for people, and I feel like a total failure. Every day, I show people what a healthy life I lead, but in truth, I can't seem to deal with my own overeating habit. It's embarrassing for me to admit that I really struggle with this.

Sharing the Struggle

I share a bit of both with my readers. At first, I only talked about the successes. But the more I blogged, I realized that I connected with my readers more by showing them that I am a real person who is relatable—someone who has similar struggles. I want to be a role model, but at the same time, I'm not perfect and I don't want people to think that I try to be. So, after about a year of blogging, I started to open up more in my posts about overeating and gaining weight after losing it.

In situations like this, I don't resent the blog or consider stopping. Blogging about my experiences also helps me deal with my issues and gives me a new perspective. My readers are always willing to leave a comment or suggestion on my blog about their experience or words of advice that help motivate and inspire me to keep on trucking along with my goals. Sometimes I write about my struggles just so I can hear what they have to say. It's nice hearing so many different points of view; it helps me get through whatever I am struggling with. I think my readers also appreciate the conversation in the comment section of my blog because it helps them too.

My Tips to Avoid Overeating

I eat enough during the day. I've noticed that if I don't eat substantial meals that include fiber-packed carbs, low-fat protein, and healthy fats, I usually encounter crazy cravings later. Now I make sure that all of my meals and snacks include a combination of all three.

I keep "trigger foods" out of the house (most of the time). Cookies, chocolate, and cereal are foods that give me trouble when it comes to portion size. Instead of keeping my favorite foods in the house, I purchase them only once in a while. I love peanut butter chips, but I buy them only every other month or so because I know I will finish off the bag in less than a week. Every now and then, it's okay, but I don't let myself have these treats in the house on a regular basis. When it comes to cereal, I buy mostly "healthy" cereal that I tend not to overdo it with. Kashi is one thing; Frosted Mini-Wheats are another!

I try not to mistake thirst for hunger. In the afternoon, especially right after lunch, I always feel hungry. But much of the time, my hunger pangs are satisfied with a big swig of water or a hot mug of tea. A little hydration goes a long way when it comes to dealing with emotional eating.

I eat by the clock. If I just ate a meal or a snack, I will try to wait at least 20 minutes before I eat something else. When I wait, I put a buffer between myself and the food, which helps make the temptation go away—at least most of the time!

I try not to be too hard on myself. A single slipup isn't going to cause me to gain pounds. If I do overdo it, I don't let it become an excuse to continue to eat poorly, though. I don't get down on myself, and I make sure to get back on track the very next time I eat.

I just don't start. Especially, when it comes to baking, I don't let myself taste my treats until it's time to do so. If I bake muffins for breakfast the night before, I don't allow myself to have one until the next morning. Same goes for cookies or blondies—I wait until dessert time. Otherwise, I'll start eating them and not stop. If I pick a specific time to enjoy a muffin or cookie, I savor it during that set period and cut myself off after that.

Damage Control

After my muffin binge, I head to the gym for my usual morning workout and run for 45 minutes on the treadmill while watching TV and listening to my iPod. I briefly think about the muffins and the caloric "damage" that I've done, but the thought soon slips out of my mind as I challenge myself to sprinting intervals on the treadmill. I alternate three minutes of steady jogging with two minutes of faster intervals—each time increasing the sprint-interval pace. I get faster and faster as the workout progresses. My body warms up, and the music on my iPod motivates me to pick up the pace. What's on my iPod right now? "California Gurls"by Katy Perry; "Paper Planes" by MIA; "Break Your Heart" by Taio Cruz; and "Bad Romance" by Lady Gaga.

By the end of the 45 minutes, I'm a sweaty mess. I feel great. The thought of eating five muffins doesn't even bother me anymore. I felt guilty after eating a fifth muffin, but that feeling is long gone. I feel energized and motivated. Exercise makes everything better.

I feel accomplished, like I did something good for my body after doing something "bad" to it by eating too many muffins. After a workout I feel confident and proud of my body. Seeing what my body can do—running five miles, for instance—makes eating too many muffins not seem so bad anymore.

Keep On Truckin'

It would have been easy for me to get down on myself about indulging in five muffins, especially knowing that I probably consumed more than half of my daily calories in just one sitting. In the past, I probably would have thrown in the towel and just kept eating those muffins until they were all gone. Instead, I refocus and just keep on truckin'.

Overeating isn't the end of the world. I've definitely had moments when I feel like I can't stop eating. I'm not sure why this happens, but I'm working on healthy ways to deal with it, like exercise. Exercise, for instance, makes me feel good about myself. It gives me confidence. After a tough workout, I'm usually proud of what my body can do. Eating one too many muffins is insignificant in comparison, which makes dealing with this sort of scenario so much easier.

If I overeat at breakfast, it doesn't mean that I continue this trend all day long. Without giving the muffins a second thought, I make sure lunch is a superhealthy meal. I don't necessarily cut calories, but I do make sure to amp up the nutritional profile of lunch with lots of fresh produce, whole grains, and some low-fat protein. An all-around nutritious and satisfying meal is the best way to get me back on track.

One slipup in my diet doesn't mean that I've fallen off the wagon for good. Living a healthy lifestyle is a commitment that I made to myself for the long haul. I know overeating and indulgences are going to happen from time to time, so I make sure to be realistic about how and what I eat and to plan accordingly when faced with a situation when I may overdo it.

Food as Art

Thankfully, I've made some great blog friends who are skilled photographers and have helped me learn how to take good shots of my food. I have a whole slew of colorful and fun plates and dishes that I use to serve my food. I often buy new ones at yard sales and Goodwill. I don't need a whole set of dishes; usually just one unique dish will do the trick when it comes to snapping a photo of my meal. I don't do too much to "style" my food, but I do make sure it looks appetizing. I'll take a lot more photos of a bright, colorful salad and put them on my blog than I do of a piece of brown, boring meatloaf. I definitely get inspiration and ideas from other blogs and magazines like *Real Simple*, which always have delicious-looking photos. Most days, I take fifty to sixty photos of my food, but, only about twenty end up on my blog. It's crazy to think how many images I take of my food!

Here are a few of my favorite muffin recipes. If you must overdo it from time to time, at least you'll know that these are filled with good ingredients.

PUMPKIN MUFFINS

The infamous pumpkin muffins! They're subtly sweet, soft, and delicious. I bet you can't eat just one!

1 cup all-purpose flour

1 cup oats

1/2 cup packed brown sugar

1 teaspoon baking powder

1/2 teaspoon baking soda

11/4 cup canned pumpkin

1 egg

1 tablespoon canola oil

1/2 teaspoon ground cinnamon

1/4 cup raisins

1/4 cup chopped walnuts

1/4 cup pumpkin seeds (to sprinkle on top of the muffins)

Preheat the oven to 375°F. Coat a muffin tin with nonstick cooking spray or line with paper muffin cups.

Combine all the ingredients in a mixing bowl, and blend well. Pour the batter evenly into the muffin cups, and bake for 20 to 22 minutes. Sprinkle a few pumpkin seeds on top of each muffin. Transfer the muffins to a rack and allow to cool. Split, spread with butter if desired, and enjoy!

MAKES 12 MUFFINS

EASY APPLE CINNAMON MUFFINS

If you've never used instant oatmeal before, this little recipe will convince you to start right now.

---

5 packets of apple-cinnamon instant oatmeal

1/4 cup all-purpose flour

1 teaspoon baking powder

2 eggs

1/4 cup canola oil

Preheat the oven to 350°F. Coat a mini-muffin tin with nonstick cooking spray. Combine all ingredients in a large mixing bowl, and blend well. Pour the batter evenly into the muffin cups, and bake for 15 to 20 minutes. Transfer the muffins to a rack and allow to cool.

MAKES 12 MINI-MUFFINS

9

HAPPY HOUR

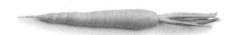

L et me be the first to say it: I'm not one to pass up a cocktail, especially at the end of a long week. A cold beer or a glass of deep red wine help to make the stresses of the week fade away. What can I say? I've been known to drink every now and then—and I have the stories to prove it!

This is not to say that I condone binge drinking. I went to college and had a great time, so more than once I've had a little too much fun and woke up with a killer hangover. I've been drunk plenty of times, but never so much that I can't control myself or don't remember the night before. I'm actually really responsible when I drink and very aware of who is driving home and which of my friends has had enough. I try to remain capable of making good decisions . . . well, most of the time!

A Wake-up Call

Three times a year, Boston's Harpoon Brewery holds a beer festival called Harpoonfest. A few years ago I had a little too much fun at one of their summer events. I was having a blast: the weather was perfect, I was talking to friends (and probably some people I didn't know very well), and the beers just kept going down! Before I knew it, I must have drunk four or five beers, which is just too much for me.

I love taking photos for *Carrots 'N' Cake*, so just the week before, Mal had given me a brand-new point-and-shoot camera for my birthday. It was the nicest camera, and I was so excited to have it. I wore the camera strap around my wrist for easy access at Harpoonfest and took lots of pictures.

Suddenly, while I was pointing something out to a friend, my camera dropped straight into Mal's full glass of beer. Tipsy as I was, I barely realized what had happened. Mal pulled my camera from his glass and, needless to say, I had killed it. I felt so terrible about ruining Mal's gift, but there was no way I'd ask him for another one. There I was at the store a few days later, purchasing the same exact model. Happy birthday to me!

The majority of my drinking episodes are not that eventful. Most of the time, I don't have more than two or three drinks over the course of an evening. When I do go out for drinks with friends, I have a great time, but I also try to keep my health in mind. I always avoid high-calorie, frozen, whipped cream–topped drinks like piña coladas, but even one too many glasses of wine can add unnecessarily to my calorie count—and doing this week after week can easily pack on the pounds! I've learned that happy hour can still be pretty healthy if I have a strategy.

Think Before You Drink

It's five thirty PM on a Friday evening, and I've just met Mal and a few of our friends at a bar downtown. Even before I walked into the bar, I mentally prepared my game plan for the evening. It's so much easier to think clearly before I've had a few adult beverages!

As my resolution for the New Year in 2009, I set a goal to limit my alcoholic drinks to three per night—no exceptions allowed. Of course, I try to have fewer than three cocktails, but that number is my absolute max. I set this number on New Year's Day after a rough night of drinking—playing beer pong with champagne is not a good idea! Needless to say, I woke up feeling terrible the next morning and vowed never to drink again. Well, most people would probably make that promise to themselves after waking up with the worst hangover of their life, but I knew that I needed a more realistic approach to drinking, especially since having a drink with friends was such a big part of my social life. I didn't want to miss out on the fun, but I knew I needed a plan.

At happy hour, it's easy for me to enjoy one drink, then another—and before I know it, I've had five cocktails. Having had that much to drink, it's really tough to turn down a slice of pizza or a sausage with peppers and onions from the street vendor on my way home. Plus, I typically wake up feeling horrible and totally unmotivated the next morning. If I remind myself to stick to three drinks before the night even begins, it's so much easier not to lose my resolve when the shots of Patrón come out!

Water First

With my mental game plan set, I take a minute to settle into the scene. Instead of making a beeline for the bar, I chat with Mal and our friends before ordering a drink. If I don't consider what I want to drink, I don't always end up making the best decision. I don't like to waste money, so I drink whatever I order even if it's not what I really want. I order a glass of ice water to sip while my friends enjoy their first cocktail. My glass of water is all part of my strategy to prevent a hangover.

We're at a bar with a really laid-back vibe. No one in our group seems to be in the mood for a crazy night, so there's no need to waste my calories by putting on my drinking shoes. My friends stay with their first round of cocktails for about thirty minutes. By then, I've eased into the evening and I'm ready to place my order: a glass of Chardonnay. I pick the most expensive glass on the list because I know that I'm more likely to sip slowly and enjoy a quality glass of wine.

If I order a cocktail or beer, it's easy to drink it quickly and order another. Wine, however, has become my go-to drink because I know I'll take my time and enjoy it. Plus, splurging on a fancy glass of wine makes me feel more sophisticated, which prevents me from guzzling it down. If I choose whatever alcohol takes me the longest to drink,

I wind up saving calories by passing on a second round. If I've already splurged earlier in the day, I'll alternate a glass of wine with a glass of water to slow my pace.

My first glass of wine is delicious—exactly what I wanted. I sip it slowly, chat with friends, and enjoy myself at Happy Hour. When my husband orders another beer, he asks me if I'd like another glass of wine. I'm only halfway through my first drink, so I decline. A little while later, though, I find myself a few sips away from the bottom of my wineglass when a friend offers to buy me my second drink of the night. I can't turn down a friendly offer like that, so I thank him and accept another glass of Chardonnay. Usually, I think through my drink order, but this time, I'm forced to make a quick decision. I like the Chardonnay a lot, so it made ordering another a lot easier.

Glass number two of Chardonnay comes and goes. I'm feeling more relaxed, a little buzzed, and I'm having a great time. The stress of the workweek has totally dissipated. I think I should just quit drinking for the night, but it doesn't look like my husband or my friends want to leave anytime soon. They're having a blast, too. I don't like to be a party pooper, so I order my third drink of the night and continue the merriment with my friends.

I don't always order drink number three. Usually, I'll have two and call it a night. That third drink is just a buffer for when I really want it, but it always makes me think twice about where the night is going. Happy hour on this particular Friday didn't seem like it would turn into a late night, but the friendly conversation and atmosphere definitely called for a third drink, which I enjoyed greatly.

Greek Life

I haven't always been so controlled with my drinking. In college and even after college, I drank like a fish. Almost every Friday and Saturday night was devoted to getting drunk, which ultimately led to consuming way too many calories. But, surprisingly, I didn't gain weight until after college, which was likely because I ate only two meals a day and I ran, which definitely helped too. I never ate breakfast, and lunch and dinner were almost always a big salad with chicken or a ham sandwich with cheese, lettuce, and tomato. The booze calories didn't catch up with me because I was barely consuming enough calories for the day!

I didn't eat this way intentionally—it's not like I was trying to lose weight. Between school, a work-study job, a part-time job waitressing, sorority responsibilities, a boyfriend, and a social life, I just didn't have time to eat well. As much as I enjoyed food, it just wasn't on my mind. I ate to live; I didn't live to eat. Oh, how things have changed!

I went to a very small, liberal arts college in upstate New York. With not much to do off campus, the on-campus scene included a social life that revolved around Greek life and drinking. You could find a party almost every night of the week where you could join in the drinking. I was part of a sorority, so I had plenty of connections to get drunk almost whenever I wanted. Greek life made it so easy.

When it wasn't midterms or finals, I'd get drunk at least twice a week on Fridays and Saturdays, and if my workload wasn't too heavy, I'd go out on Wednesday nights, too. Usually, the evening would start pretty tamely, with a few cocktails at a party. Theme parties were big at my college, so the parties would typically be really festive and fun, which always led me to drink more. Plus, the alcohol was "free." My sorority dues helped pay for the parties.

Most nights, my sorority sisters and I would drink well into the night as we hopped from party to party around campus. The evening would end up with a foodfest when we got back to the dorm. My go-to postdrinking snack was Easy Mac. It was fast, quick, and cheesy—perfect for a girl who'd had too much to drink. I remember that one night I ate at least three packages in one sitting. (Just the thought of it now turns my stomach.)

Over the years, this late-night eating has occurred pretty much anytime I got drunk. I've downed chicken fingers, pizza, Chinese food, a grilled cheese sandwich—pretty much anything fatty and greasy. Much of the time, it's food that I wouldn't normally eat if I were sober. But when I am drunk and hungry, I'll eat whatever seems appetizing without a second thought—and I almost always regret my decision. I either feel terrible about myself before I go to bed or wake up the next morning and vow to never engage in late-night drunk snacking. Usually, a workout or healthy breakfast made me feel better, but overdoing it like that never helped me get ahead when it came to reducing calories and losing weight, especially after college.

I set the three-drink rule for myself in early 2009, and I've done a great job sticking to it. It puts me in control of a situation where I could easily lose control. In college and my early twenties, I could easily polish off eight drinks in a night, which was extremely damaging to my body. Now that

I'm older (and wiser), I realize that I can no longer treat my body this way. It doesn't appreciate this type of treatment and lets me know! The three-drink rule has definitely slowed my pace when it comes to drinking and going out to the bars—and that makes sense for my lifestyle, too.

My Tips for Lower-calorie Drinks

Instead of a Margarita: High-quality tequila, like Patrón Silver, with seltzer, lime juice, and splash of Diet Sprite. Tastes so close to the real thing!

Instead of a Cape Codder: Raspberry-flavored vodka with seltzer. Flavored vodkas impart a lot of flavor without a lot of calories.

Instead of a Cosmopolitan: Orange-flavored vodka with seltzer and a splash of cranberry juice. Pour it into a martini glass, and you'll never know the difference.

Order seltzer: By ordering seltzer for your first drink and then a cocktail when your friends are on their second round, you'll save 100 to 200 calories before the night even really begins! And think twice about fruit juice—it's a high-calorie mixer.

WHITE SANGRIA

This is one of my favorite cocktails to serve at summer parties. It's a crowd-pleaser and so easy to make. Plus, it's relatively low in calories and contains nutritious berries.

1 1/2 liters dry white wine
1/2 liter soda water
1/2 liter diet citrus soda (like Fresca)
1 (8 ounce) bag frozen berries

Combine the wine, soda water, and citrus soda in a large pitcher; then add the frozen berries. Chill the sangria for approximately 45 minutes in the refrigerator. Serve in your favorite glass, and enjoy!

MAKES ABOUT 8 SERVINGS

PIMM'S CUP

The next time you have friends over, try this fruity punch made with Pimm's No. 1. The Brits serve it throughout the hot summer months, and I really think they're on to something.

1/2 cup freshly squeezed lemon juice

1/2 cup freshly squeezed lime juice

1/2 cup freshly squeezed orange juice

1/2 cup Simple Syrup (page 106)

1/2 cup Pimm's No. 1

    Ice cubes

    2-inch center chunk of an unpared European cucumber, thinly sliced crosswise into 6 rounds

12 fresh mint leaves

    About 2 cups chilled tonic water

Combine the lemon, lime, and orange juices with the syrup and Pimm's in a pitcher, and stir to blend. Place a few ice cubes in each of 6 tall glasses, along with a cucumber slice and 2 mint leaves. Add the Pimm's mixture, dividing equally and to at most 2 inches from the top. Top off each glass with tonic water.

MAKES ABOUT 6 DRINKS

SIMPLE SYRUP

Lots of cocktails start with this simple sugar-water syrup. Any leftovers can be stored in the fridge.

---

2 cups sugar

1½ cups water

Combine the sugar and water in a small saucepan, and heat to boiling over medium-high heat, stirring to dissolve the sugar. Boil 1 minute, remove from the heat, and let stand until cool.

MAKES ABOUT 2 ½ CUPS

MARGARITA GRANITA

Tequila all around! Serve this refreshing treat at your next summer party, and please everyone.

3¼ cups water

1 cup sugar

3 limes, zested and juiced

1 orange, zested and juiced

3 tablespoons tequila

Combine the water, sugar, and zests (not the juices!) in a medium saucepan, and heat to boiling over medium heat, stirring until the sugar dissolves. Boil for 2 minutes; then set aside to steep until cool.

When the sugar mixture is cool, add the juices through a sieve; then add the tequila. Mix until blended; then pour into an 11- by 9-inch glass baking dish. Freeze until frozen, about 3 hours, stirring occasionally.

To serve, let the granita stand a few minutes at room temperature to soften slightly; if it is hard-frozen, break the granita into chunks and process in a food processor until icy but not slushy. Scrape into short glasses with a fork to make crystals.

MAKES ABOUT 10 SERVINGS

10

GIRL STUFF

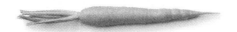

It's Saturday night, and I'm headed to my friend Beth's house for a girls' night— complete with cocktails and appetizers. Beth is a great cook and always goes above and beyond when it comes to entertaining, so even before I get into my car to drive to her house, I know that I need to practice some self-control at her get-together.

Beth is someone I have known most of my life, but we didn't become good friends until recently. I hadn't seen her for a few weeks, so on this particular night I was looking forward to catching up with her, sipping cocktails, and spending time with some of our other friends.

This is the type of social occasion I used to fear. Surrounded by good friends and wrapped up in the festivities, I found it so easy to overindulge in both food and drink. Then I'd spend the next day feeling miserable and disappointed in myself. Now, after some practice and a little trial and error, I've learned that social settings don't have to be a free-for-all when it comes to eating and drinking. At Beth's girls' night, I made sure to keep the night healthy and had fun at the same time.

Assess the Situation

When I arrive at Beth's house, I take a moment to soak in the atmosphere instead of making a beeline for the bar or the buffet. Beth has greeted me warmly at the door, so I get a feel for the room, preview the food spread, and take a peek at the cocktail selection before I actually select anything to eat or drink. I know if I start to indulge at the first plate of food I see, I'm only setting myself up for disaster. Instead I take a moment to figure out what I really want and ultimately make healthier choices.

There are already a few women huddled around the food table and sipping on colorful martinis. All of the women are dressed stylishly with form-fitting pants, high heels, and colorful tops. I'm glad that I decided on the outfit that I did: dark trouser jeans, round-toe black heels, and a silky teal top. I always stress about what to wear to these types of events, but I'm happy with my outfit. I feel upbeat and confident as I settle into the party.

Beth immediately offers me a cocktail from the bar. As we know, I like to enjoy a cocktail or two, but without a preset limit, I find it difficult to turn down a third or fourth glass once I've had a couple of drinks. And alcohol also lowers my inhibitions about eating high-calorie foods. So, well before the night begins, I determine how many cocktails I will have and stick to that number.

At the bar, I see that Beth has prepared a number of cocktails ahead of time in large pitchers, so guests can easily help themselves to a mixed drink. Beth has created three special cocktails for the evening: Cosmopolitan, Lemon Drop, and Flirtini. The Flirtini is a mix of vodka, Triple Sec, pineapple juice, and champagne, and the combination of ingredients immediately grabs my attention. Before I know it, Beth is chilling a martini glass and pouring me one. Just like that, I have a refreshing, sweet, and bubbly cocktail in my hand. Beth is clearly the hostess with the mostest. Good thing I've already decided to drink just one cocktail tonight—Beth mixes a strong cocktail. I take my time and sip slowly.

Once I have a drink in my hand, I walk over and say hello to the women huddled near the buffet. I know most of the ladies at girls' night, but Beth makes sure to introduce me to those I have never met. I meet one of Beth's college friends and her cousin. Both women are outgoing and friendly, and we immediately hit it off with our similar interests in cooking and baking.

After a little chatting, it's time to check out the food options. Beth always makes the most delicious foods when she entertains, and I skipped dinner just so I could indulge in some of her delicious party foods. But now I'm starving, so just a few sips of Flirtini are starting to go straight to my head.

I exercised during the day before Beth's party because I knew I was going to splurge that night. I also made sure to eat two well-balanced meals for breakfast and lunch, so I didn't show up starving to her party that night. On days like this, I try to eat meals that are packed with fibrous carbs, protein, and a little bit of fat, which keeps me buzzing along all day. I'm less likely to snack, so I save those calories for my splurge in the evening.

Smart Choices

When it comes to higher-calorie party fare, my rule is this: If it's not healthy and I can make it myself, I don't try it. So I pass on the plate of cheese, pepperoni slices, and crackers but go right for the bites of panini of smoked turkey, brie, sliced apples, and mango chutney. The combination of flavors sounds unique, and the ingredients are mostly healthy, so I grab one right away. All of the flavors blend incredibly well, and the multigrain bread is slightly seasoned, thick, and grilled to perfection.

After eating a panini, my taste buds are awake and want something more to eat. I could easily eat those panini all night long, but instead I take a minute to prepare a small plate of food for myself instead of snacking all night on appetizers. This provides me with a visual account of how much I am eating. It's easy for me to lose track of small bites here and there over the course of the night, especially in a fun and lively atmosphere. I could have easily eaten a whole plate of those delicious panini bites without even realizing it, so my plate system really works for me. And I can always go back for a refill if I'm still hungry.

By the end of the night, my stomach is full and my martini glass is empty. I've spent the entire night catching up with friends and laughing a lot. I've learned that when I turn my focus away from the foods and drink and to my friends, it makes it so much easier to resist the temptation of party food. I had a ton of fun at girls' night and I woke up feeling good about my party decisions the next morning.

Self-Confidence

For the greater part of my life, an evening like this would have been difficult for me. I've always had self-confidence issues. Reading my blog, one would probably never guess that I struggled with how I felt about myself. As I mentioned earlier, my family was really poor, so I never had the most stylish clothing and I couldn't do all of the fun things that my friends could do. We just didn't have the money to spend on family vacations, trips to the amusement park, or even meals out at restaurants. I always felt like I wasn't as "cool" as the other kids.

I went through almost my entire life feeling this way—even in high school and college I felt like I didn't quite fit in with my group of friends. In college, for instance, I belonged to a sorority, so I had a huge network of "sisters" that were supposedly my friends. I'm not saying that I didn't like these women or they didn't like me, but I always questioned if they really liked me and accepted me as part of their group. From the outside, it probably looked like I had a ton of friends, but really, I felt a true friendship with only a handful of them.

This lack of self-confidence plagued me until my mid-twenties, when I finally started to come out of my shell. I have always been an introvert, but this time in my life really allowed me to put myself out there, meet people, and develop my true self. The most important part of feeling confident was feeling good about the way my body looked.

From a young age, I was cursed with a large chest on a petite body. All of the women on my mother's side of the family are built the same way. While some women would love to be well-endowed, I hated it. A large chest made me constantly self-conscious and especially uncomfortable when it came to physical activity like running or playing soccer. Wearing two sports bras while the other gals on my soccer team wore one was always embarrassing, and dance recitals with shoulder-baring costumes were always a challenge. I even had to buy a specially made bra to wear with my senior prom dress. Basically, having a big chest was more of a pain in the butt than a blessing.

Over the years, my big chest bothered me, but I never thought I could do anything about it. I just figured it was something that I had to live with. But then a friend of mine decided to get a breast reduction. She looked great after the surgery—and she was so happy! So, of course, I had a million questions for her about the operation itself, the costs, and recovery. It turns out that her surgery was covered by her health insurance and the recovery time was just two weeks. As soon as I talked to her, I started making plans to have the procedure. I didn't have a single qualm about my decision.

I visited my primary care doctor and told her what I wanted to have done. Turns out that I was more than qualified to have my health insurance cover the costs of my surgery. (My co-pay for the whole thing was just twenty-five dollars.)

The day of the surgery, I wasn't nervous at all. I was excited! I couldn't wait to have a smaller, perkier chest that didn't prevent me from exercising or wearing the cute tops that I wanted to wear. I was more than ready for the surgery. My mother and Mal were not, however. They were worried sick for the duration of the nearly six-hour operation. They still crack jokes about what I said to the surgeon when I woke up in the recovery room: "That was quick!" The surgeon was exhausted, but he just smiled at my ridiculous statement.

During surgery, the doctor removed more than a pound of breast tissue from each breast, which was required for my health insurance to cover the surgery. I was more than happy to reduce my cup size from a G to a D. I woke up groggy and sore, but I was so glad that the surgery was over and that I would have a chest size more appropriate for my body.

After the bandages came off and the swelling went down, I instantly loved my new body. I looked "normal" for once! I didn't have guys constantly staring at my chest, and I could finally wear cute bras instead of the old-lady ones that I was forced to wear. As far as body confidence went, I did a complete 180 and had a ton of it! I had the surgery done right when I started to lose weight, and it definitely jump-started my motivation to continue toward my goal weight. It also gave me the body confidence to do so.

MEEGHAN'S EDAMAME GUACAMOLE

My cousin Meeghan made this for a family party, and I've been obsessed with it ever since. It's now something I make for Mal and myself whenever the mood strikes.

1 ripe avocado

1 cup shelled edamame

1 lime, juiced

1 chipotle pepper in adobo sauce (these are really hot, so use at your discretion)

2 teaspoons minced garlic

1/3 bunch of cilantro, chopped

1/2 cup chopped tomato

1/4 cup chopped onion

Salt

Pepper

Combine all ingredients in a food processor, adding salt and pepper to taste, until smooth. Serve cold with pita chips, tortilla chips, or crackers.

MAKES ABOUT 2 CUPS

FRESH ONION DIP

Everyone loves the sour cream and French onion soup mix recipe for potato chip dip. This is something altogether different. Veggies and pita are best with this.

---

1 cup unsalted dry-curd cottage cheese

1/3 cup skim milk

2 teaspoons fresh lemon juice

1 teaspoon onion powder

1/2 teaspoon garlic powder

1/4 cup finely chopped green onion

Combine the cheese, milk, lemon juice, onion powder, and garlic powder in a food processor, and process until smooth. Scrape into a bowl, and fold in the green onion. Cover and refrigerate at least 1 hour to allow the flavors to blend.

MAKES ABOUT 1¼ CUPS

GREEN AND RED NACHOS

Bet you can't eat just one of these! Not to worry. Each one is only 28 calories, so it doesn't really matter.

42 large low-fat baked tortilla chips

1 pint cherry tomatoes, diced

1/2 cup chopped green onion

1 (8-ounce) package shredded reduced-fat Mexican
     cheese blend

Preheat the oven to 450°F. Arrange the tortilla chips in a single layer on 2 parchment paper–lined baking sheets and sprinkle each with tomatoes, green onion, and cheese. Bake until the cheese melts, 4 to 5 minutes.

MAKES 42 NACHOS

11

THE COOKIE SWAP

A cookie swap is a chance for a bunch of people to bake their favorite type of cookie and then swap their cookies for some of everyone else's. During the event, you taste a bunch of cookies, and at the end of the event, you take home a whole slew of cookies to enjoy at a later date. Of course, the idea of a cookie swap always sounds like a great idea to me, so when my friend Shannon invited me to one for a bunch of Boston-area food bloggers, I accepted her invitation without hesitation. I did, however, plan my day accordingly. I ate a light breakfast and lunch and hit the gym for a sweaty workout to get a head start on the cookie calories that I was about to consume. I had good intentions for keeping my day healthy and not going overboard in the calorie department.

The night before, however, I really overdid it while making my treat for the party: Butterscotch Chocolate Chip Bars. I sampled the batter quite a few times and then later the actual baked treat. In fact, I ate so many bars, I felt sick to my stomach and had to cancel dinner plans with my friend Jen. I couldn't even fathom the thought of a meal out. I felt like a five-year-old child who had eaten too much candy and now had a bellyache. It was not my finest moment explaining to my friend that I had eaten too many cookies and had to cancel our evening out. Thankfully, she was understanding and we hung out at my apartment for a couple of hours and just chatted instead of eating dinner together. Even though it worked out, I was pretty embarrassed.

Losing Control

When it was time for the cookie swap, I tried to keep my cool with the food, but it was quite a spread. Beyond the cookies, there were so many delicious options to choose from—fresh salsa and guacamole, coconut-chai almonds, salmon mousse dip, bacon-flavored potato chips. Instead of forgoing the appetizers and saving my calories for the main event, I ended up trying all of the food and continuing to sample it until it was time to swap.

By the time the cookie swap began, I was already feeling full from all of the food I had just eaten. I'm sure it was all in my head, but I swear my pants felt tighter and my thighs grew! At that point, I should have known to lay off sampling the cookies. The whole point was to swap cookies to take home with you for later. I didn't need to eat them all at the event.

So Many Cookies

But I couldn't help myself. There were so many delicious options: Break-Up Bars, which tasted like Twix bars with thick caramel, chocolate, and cookie; Peanut Butter Bars with chocolate and pretzels on top and Whoppers inside; Chocolate-Covered Cookie Dough Truffles. I had no chance resisting these goodies. My willpower around this type of food is zero.

I'm not shy about my love for desserts, especially cookies, so I dug right in. I started with a Break-Up Bar and went for a small piece to help pace myself. It tasted so delicious. As soon as I took that first bite, I knew that I needed more. I also knew that it might be difficult to stop myself. Then I ate a Peanut Butter Bar, two Chocolate Crinkle Cookies, two Cookie Dough Truffles, a Maple Bacon Toffee Oatmeal Cookie, a Lemon Almond Cranberry Crescent, and even one of my own Butterscotch Chocolate Chip Bars, as if I hadn't had enough of them already!

Before I knew it, I had tried almost every single cookie at the event. I'm not sure if the other bloggers noticed, but I definitely had my share of treats for the afternoon. Initially, I didn't feel embarrassed. It was a special event and we had all made delectable treats to share with one another. I thought it was okay to overindulge. But after eating close to ten cookies, I knew that I had eaten too much. Plus, all of those cookies were starting to settle into my stomach, and I didn't feel very well.

Time to Go

I ended up being one of the first people to leave. I didn't want to be tempted any longer by all of the cookies at the party, so I thought it would be best to just avoid the situation altogether. I had lost control, my stomach hurt because I had eaten so much, I was embarrassed that everyone saw me pig out on cookies, and I knew that I would continue to chow down on cookies if I didn't leave soon.

I was depressed on my ride home. I had planned a splurge into my day—I ate lightly and exercised before-hand—but I really overdid it. I was terribly frustrated that I had lost control, and maybe I should have known that a get-together like this would be trouble for me. At the same time, I didn't want to admit to myself that I couldn't control my appetite around sweet treats. I almost felt hopeless about the situation.

When I got home that evening, I gave myself a little pep talk. I blog three times a day about what I eat, and I give people all over the world advice about healthy living. If I couldn't get it together, people would see me as a hypocrite. Sure, I didn't blog that I ate a zillion cookies at the cookie swap, but *I* knew that I ate that many, and, of course, so did my body. Even though those cookie calories didn't show up on my blog, my body still knew they were there.

After my little pity party, I vowed to document every single morsel that I ate on my blog. That way, I'd be accountable when I ate ten cookies in one sitting. Plus, it would make me think twice when reaching for a second or third or even fourth treat. Would I really want to document another piece of cake and display it on the blog? This tactic actually worked, and I became much more open about my dessert "problem" to my blog readers.

My readers responded really well, and since then I've written quite a bit more about my overeating issue when it comes to baked goods and other treats. A lot of people seem to identify with me. I think my readers find it comforting—perhaps even inspiring—that a "healthy living" blogger also has the same struggles but manages to deal with them and live a mostly healthy lifestyle. Readers also ask me for my advice with how to deal with overeating. I haven't quite dealt with it myself, but I am learning what works for me, and I enjoy sharing my experience with other people because it may just help them too.

The Sweet Tooth Wins

When it comes to maintaining my healthy lifestyle, and especially my weight, it's easy to step it up with more intense workouts or an extra trip to the gym to help balance out the extra calories that I consume from goodies like baked goods and other treats. But when it comes to my eating habits, my sweet tooth reigns supreme. It's tough for me to turn down my favorite treats.

Even so, I also know that the calories that I burn through exercise will never equal the cookie calories that I consume. I love exercise and fitness, but I'm not obsessive about it. Most of my workouts are 60 minutes or less, which means that even the hardest, sweatiest workout won't burn the calories that I've consumed if I'm not careful. Plus, I don't really have time to spend all day in the gym, and even if I did, I'd likely get bored. If I go out for a run, I'll sometimes run for more than 60 minutes, but my long runs are only once a month or so (unless I am training for a road race).

A few weeks after the cookie swap, a light bulb went off in my head: Almost every time I overindulge in sweets, it's when they are available in large portions, like a batch of freshly baked cookies, a pint of Malted Milk Ball Gelato, or a cookie swap. When the sweets are just sitting around, especially at home, I just can't say no—and I almost always go back for seconds, and even thirds.

However, when I dine out, I can usually talk myself out of ordering a ten-dollar dessert, especially when I'm paying for it. I almost always enjoy an entrée and a cocktail, so it's easy to turn down the waiter's offer to see the dessert menu when the time comes. The act of ordering a dessert makes me stop and think, so I can decide if I really want a sweet treat at the end of the meal. At home or at parties, I don't have this time buffer to slow down my actions. I just reach for dessert without a second thought. Since the food is available, I feel like I have no reason to not go back for another serving. Of course I know that I'm consuming more calories than I need to, but the accessibility of the food doesn't seem to affect the satisfaction of my sweet tooth.

I would never give up dessert completely, so moving forward, I decided to implement a few rules to help me get my portion sizes in control, which would help me and hopefully show my blog readers that you can have your cake and eat it too—without overdoing it!

My Healthy Tips for Dessert Control

I enjoy a small treat every day. If I don't allow myself my favorite goodies, I am more likely to overdo it. It's like a mini–Cookie Friday every day.

I find a five-minute distraction. Before reaching for another cookie, I try to find something to distract my sweet tooth—like checking my e-mail, painting my nails, or running a quick errand. Getting my mind off dessert is the key to preventing overindulging at home.

I consider the consequences. Reminding myself that this treat will end up on my blog for the world to see helps me turn down more dessert than I need!

Changing my "bad" dessert habits hasn't been easy. It's not like I stopped enjoying dessert overnight. I still love (and crave) cookies, cake, and ice cream, but now I view them differently. Instead of being a staple in my diet, I try to see dessert as a special treat. I still have it every day, but I make sure that when I choose to eat such a goodie, it's a somewhat nutritious option and I keep my portion size small. For this reason, I've started to bake my own yummy treats at home, but in small batches.

I started baking my own desserts at home—cookies, sweet breads, blondies—but I'd inevitably end up eating the whole batch within a day or two. Having those freshly baked goods sitting around my house was constant temptation that I would indulge in multiple times a day. Controlling what went into my baked goods made me feel better about indulging in them. A homemade pumpkin bar made with shredded coconut and dates was a much better option than a store-bought cookie with saturated fat and hard-to-pronounce ingredients.

Small Batches are Key

However, when I found myself eating a pumpkin bar before I even poured my morning cup of coffee, I knew that I couldn't keep full batches of baked goods in the house. I'd just eat them until they were all gone. So, from that point on, I started to make small batches of my baking experiments—a smaller pan became my new favorite baking tool. I made only enough batter to fill it, which resulted in about a dozen or even half dozen treats, which was a much more reasonable amount to have sitting around the house constantly tempting me. Even if I ate a half dozen oatmeal raisin cookies, it wasn't a full batch. Basically, baking less was the portion control that I needed.

PUMPKIN DATE NUT BARS

It's not easy, but when I'm under control, I limit myself to one of these amazing bars a day. They stay moist for several days, and I always get Mal to help me eat them. That helps!

1/4 cup canned pumpkin

1/2 cup sugar

1 egg

1/4 cup canola oil

1/2 cup whole wheat flour

1/4 tsp baking powder

1/4 tsp salt

1/4 tsp cinnamon

3/4 cup chopped dates

1/2 cup chopped walnuts

Preheat the oven to 350°F. Spray an 8- by 8-inch baking pan with nonstick cooking spray.

In a large bowl, combine the pumpkin, sugar, egg, and oil. Sift together the flour and the baking powder, salt, and cinnamon, and add to the pumpkin mixture, stirring to combine. Stir in the dates and the walnuts.

Spread the batter in the pan, and bake for 25 to 30 minutes, until a wooden pick (or knife) inserted near the center comes out clean. Remove the pan from the oven.

Allow to cool before cutting.

MAKES 12 BARS

OATMEAL RAISIN COOKIES

Oatmeal and raisins are a favorite combination of mine, and I'm guilty of overdoing it, but I want to share these cookies with you. I'm always trying to increase the nutrition while reducing the calories in my favorite baked goods. Chickpeas have lots of fiber and some protein and add some moisture to the cookies as well.

- 1/4 cup all-purpose flour
- 1/4 cup old-fashioned oats
- 1/4 cup chickpeas
- 1/4 cup brown sugar, packed
- 1/4 cup canola oil
- 1 teaspoon vanilla extract
- Cinnamon
- 1/4 cup raisins

Preheat the oven to 350°F. Coat a baking sheet with non-stick cooking spray.

In a mini–food processor or blender, combine the flour, oats, chickpeas, brown sugar, oil, vanilla, and cinnamon to taste. Pulse until thick and smooth. Stir in the raisins. Using a tablespoon, scoop the batter onto the baking sheet, leaving 1 inch between cookies. Flatten each cookie with the bottom of the spoon. Bake for 18 to 20 minutes, until golden brown. Remove to a rack to cool before serving.

MAKES 6 (3-INCH) COOKIES

CHOCOLATE PUMPKIN LOAF

Super moist and chocolaty, this is one of my favorites with a warm cup of tea or coffee.

11/4 cups all-purpose flour

3/4 cup packed brown sugar

1/2 cup white sugar

1/4 cup unsweetened cocoa powder

2 eggs

1 teaspoon baking powder

1/2 teaspoon baking soda

1/4 teaspoon salt

2 teaspoons ground cinnamon

1/2 teaspoon grated nutmeg

1 teaspoon vanilla extract

71/2 ounces canned pumpkin

1 cup chocolate chips

Preheat the oven to 325°F. Grease a loaf pan. Combine all ingredients in a large mixing bowl, and blend well. Pour batter into loaf pan, and bake for 40 to 45 minutes, until top is firm and a toothpick comes out clean. Allow the loaf to cool for 15 minutes, and dust with powdered sugar if desired.

MAKES 1 LOAF

DOUBLE-CHOCOLATE
TEA CAKES

Here is another one of my seriously chocolate treats. Because it is so chocolaty, I usually can very happily limit myself to one.

10 ounces bittersweet chocolate, chopped

3/4 cup (1 1/2 sticks) unsalted butter, cut into 1-inch pieces

5 eggs

1/2 cup sugar

3/4 cup all-purpose flour

3/4 teaspoon baking powder

Unsweetened cocoa powder for dusting

Preheat the oven to 325°F and generously grease the cups of a regular-size muffin pan. Cut 12 rounds of parchment paper to fit the cups, and place a round in each cup.

Combine the chocolate and butter in a small saucepan, and heat over low heat, stirring frequently, until melted and smooth. Remove from the heat and set aside.

Combine the eggs and sugar in a medium bowl and beat at high speed with an electric mixer until light and fluffy, about 6 minutes. Combine the flour and baking powder in a sifter, and sift over the egg mixture. Gently fold to mix. Add the chocolate mixture and fold to mix.

CONTINUED

Pour the batter into the prepared muffin cups and bake until the tops spring back when lightly pressed with your finger, about 20 minutes.

Cool the cakes in the pan 2 minutes; then transfer to a wire rack placed over a baking sheet. Dust with cocoa sprinkled through a fine sieve.

MAKES 12 TEA CAKES

12

SUNDAYS WITH MAL

L ike many people, I live a hectic life that seems to include very little free time. Between work obligations, my husband, and my pug, I'm on the go from dawn till dusk. Some people might think that healthy living is nearly impossible when you're crazy busy, but a little planning on Sunday afternoon goes a long way for me. In fact, my little Sunday ritual has become essential to my sanity. If I don't take the time, Monday through Friday ends up being much more stressful than it really needs to be.

This Sunday morning starts with pancakes and iced coffee. My wonderful husband offers to make pancakes for the two of us. Mal doesn't cook frequently, but when he does, his meals turn out amazingly well. This morning, he gets down to business making his special recipe.

On the weekends, I like to have laid-back mornings, lounging in my pj's with an iced coffee and a big breakfast— often pancakes. Then I will go to the gym and have a light lunch to even out my morning splurge.

Pancakes and Beyond

Pancakes are just one of the many foods that my husband has reintroduced to my life. Of course, I've always liked pancakes, but I rarely ate them because they're just not a nutritious option for breakfast. They're high in calories, made with refined carbohydrates, and offer hardly any nutritional value. However, Mal thinks pancakes are easily the best breakfast ever. He'd probably eat them every morning if they didn't take so long to make.

Mal has reintroduced a whole slew of foods that I had banished from my life, including pizza, ground beef, hot dogs, and potato chips. In fact, I never even liked potato chips until we moved in together. I might have had a chip or two with some dip when I went to parties, but I never really cared for them. Chips have little nutritional value, and I'd much rather "spend" my calories on something else. Now I have a huge love for potato chips: barbeque, cheddar, salt and vinegar, sour cream and chive—I pretty much love them all.

An open bag of chips can be a dangerous situation in our house. Mal has no reason to watch what he eats. He can eat anything and not gain an ounce. He's lucky like that. So when he opens a bag of potato chips, he'll keep eating them until he's satisfied, which means he'll easily eat half the bag. This also means that I will keep going back for more—one handful after another. I can't seem to stop when Mal is enjoying potato chips by the handful too. We're enjoying them together, so I guess he's supporting my potato chip habit. I should just walk away, but sharing a bag of chips is too easy.

Overdoing it on potato chips doesn't happen every single time a bag of potato chips is taken out of the cupboard, but a lot of the time, it's tough to turn down a handful or two when my husband is sitting next to me chomping away. We're spending time together, usually sitting on the couch, so sharing a snack with him seems to fit right in, even if I'm not hungry. I know that a few chips aren't a big deal, but it becomes a problem when the two of us eat half the bag together!

Portion Control

Over the years, I've started to use a bowl to portion out a couple of servings of chips. I know I'm going to want some as soon as Mal takes out the bag, so I grab a bowl from the kitchen and fill it with chips. Once they're gone, they're gone! I rarely go back for more because a bowlful is a good visual reminder that I've already eaten a couple of servings.

Mal also likes to eat a big dinner, while I've always made breakfast my biggest meal of the day. I follow that old nutritional adage, "Eat breakfast like a king, lunch like a prince, and dinner like a pauper," and try to eat my larger meals early in the day and my smaller meals in the evening.

There are a number of reasons why this balance of meals works for me. I often exercise first thing in the morning, so I like to refuel with a big breakfast (600 to 700 calories) packed with healthy carbs and protein. I used to eat a much smaller breakfast following a morning work-out, but I would be starving by lunch. Over time, my body has gotten used to eating most of its calories in the early hours of the day. My lunch is usually a tiny bit smaller than breakfast (500 to 600 calories), with a good-size snack in the afternoon (200 to 300 calories) and, of course, occasional treats (100 to 300 calories). Eating the majority of my calories in the first part of the day keeps my energy up and my metabolism buzzing along. Dinner is often my smallest meal of the day (400 to 500 calories), which is usually made up of protein, complex carbs, and lots of veggies. Since I'm also an early riser, it makes sense for me to front-load my caloric intake. I hit the sack before ten PM and don't need a ton of calories in the later part of the day. Finally, breakfast is my favorite meal of the day, so why not start the day off right with a hearty meal of my favorite foods?

Living with a Manly Man

Mal, on the other hand, would prefer to eat the exact opposite way, with breakfast as his smallest meal and dinner as his largest. This becomes problematic for my waistline because I eat a big breakfast, followed by a medium-size lunch and a big dinner. Even though I don't have to eat large portions of the meals, it's hard for me to say no to some of his favorite dishes.

And Mal does prefer "manly" food. I'd probably eat a salad, a sandwich, or a bowl of soup every night of the week, if I could. But Mal gets bored with these options. He needs "real food," like chicken, beef, and pasta, which are foods that I enjoy but are much too heavy for me to have for dinner. As you can imagine, it's hard to turn down such delicious dinners—especially when they're the product of my own home cooking. I try my best to make the meals healthier, typically by adding lots of vegetables or a side salad, but sometimes homemade pizza wins over homemade salad.

Mal is in a great mood this morning. He dances around the kitchen, mixing pancake batter while singing along to Oasis's "Live Forever." He stops to sip his home-made iced coffee before continuing to make the batter—and scoops a spoonful of raw batter right from the bowl. I'm totally grossed out, but Mal loves his special pancake recipe, whether raw or cooked! I'm happy to see my husband enjoying his Sunday morning—and the guy is making me pancakes, so who am I to complain?

Last night was an early evening, so we woke up bright and early after a good night's sleep. I know that Mal loves waking up with the sun to get his Sunday started off on the right foot—I do too. Getting moving first thing in the morning allows us to accomplish so much more and seems to extend the length of the weekend.

Mal has already had a chance to shower, dress, and drink half of his iced coffee by the time I return from walking the dog. We work together well this way: divide and conquer. From household chores to running errands to caring for our dog, we split the tasks equally and fairly. Luckily, each of us has our own likes and dislikes that make us very compatible as a couple. For instance, Mal absolutely hates doing laundry, but I enjoy it. To me, it's an easy task that I don't mind doing. Folding laundry is actually sort of relaxing for me.

Even before we got married, everything in our relationship was divided fifty-fifty. Almost two years into married life, everything is still equally split—right down to whose turn it is to pay for dinner. I'm not saying that this ratio doesn't shift from time to time. It does, just like in any ever-evolving relationship—but our basic premise is that our relationship involves equal participation and responsibility.

Once the pancakes are cooking on the griddle, Mal stands guard, ready to flip them as soon as the batter in the middle of the pancake starts to bubble. I join Mal in the kitchen and sip the glass of iced coffee that he hands me. He has made it just the way I like it: soy milk and, of course, a straw (the stainless steel, reusable variety). I can't drink iced coffee without a straw. It's just not possible.

Mal and I try to keep our Sunday mornings laid-back and relaxing, but they never lack for a planning session. When we can, we start with a big, leisurely breakfast. Usually, it's our only day to bum around and take our time in the morning, so we like to make our first meal of the day a special occasion. Mal and I are both planners at heart, and our brains never stop thinking that way. We're always trying to maximize our time and energy, so planning our life efficiently is a top priority for us—even on a Sunday morning.

Making a List

While our pancakes cook, we discuss our day. I reel off a few things that I want to get done; then Mal acknowledges my to-do list and adds his own tasks for the day. Eventually, our list gets too long to remember, so I finally write everything down on a piece of paper, which makes it easier to formulate a plan of attack. Today's to-do list includes grocery shopping, visiting the dog park, exercising, making iced coffee, and changing the bedding.

The tasks on our combined list don't seem too difficult to accomplish, especially since almost all of them can be accomplished in one trip. The toughest is easily grocery shopping. You'd think that as a foodie, I'd love taking a trip to the grocery store, but since I wait until Sunday afternoon, it makes for a crowded and stressful shopping experience. Mal and I should probably do the grocery shopping during the workweek to save us the stress, but neither of us enjoys the task, so we typically tackle it together.

Grocery shopping is also a daunting task because I am a cheapskate. You'd think that I'd be comfortable with spending money on delicious gourmet food—and sometimes I'm okay with paying a premium price for top-quality food—but I also know when I should be saving money. In fact, saving money is always in the back of my mind, so our weekly grocery shopping always requires lots of planning and coupons.

A Well-Stocked Kitchen

My Sunday shopping planning actually starts during the week with a list of items that we have run out of or we want to buy for the next week; that list usually includes meals I want to make during the week, too. When we're out of nutritious eats, I make it a point to "put it on the list."

This list hangs on the front of our refrigerator so we can easily add to it when a thought strikes. The foods that are most nutritious are priority items on my grocery list, so I rarely, if ever, run out of oatmeal, soy milk, or bananas. I view these items as foods that do something more than just fill my stomach. They provide essential vitamins and minerals, so I want them at the top of my shopping list and always in my kitchen. I rarely forget items that we want to replenish or add to the following week's menu.

After reviewing the shopping list, I assess the current situation in the kitchen. I look to see what we already have in our cupboards, refrigerator, and freezer. Then I start to use what is already available as building blocks to plan the coming week's meals. For instance, a jar of marinated artichokes in the cupboard and shredded mozzarella and a jar of leftover pesto in the refrigerator become the basis for a pesto-artichoke pizza. A bunch of super–ripe bananas become a speedy breakfast for the workweek as they are baked into homemade banana bread. Utilizing foods that we already have available saves us money because we don't buy additional items and we don't waste what we already have.

Next, I see what types of coupons and sales are available. I keep a coupon organizer on top of our refrigerator along with our reusable grocery bags, so I won't forget them when I head to the grocery store. Each week, I clip coupons and add them to the organizer for my Sunday meal planning. The coupons and store sales help define our meals for the week. I rarely buy food items at full price. For instance, if canned black beans are on sale, they are turned into a Mexican dish. If I have a coupon for Greek yogurt, it becomes part of an easily transportable lunch for the workweek.

The biggest key to maintaining my weight and a healthy lifestyle is cooking healthy food at home—and that is only possible thanks to a well-stocked, user-friendly kitchen. If I have plenty of healthy food around, I'm more likely to eat it. I hate seeing food go to waste. Plus, finding ways to save money is sort of fun for me, so I try to save every little bit I can when grocery shopping and meal planning for the week.

For me, it's all about balance. Take dinner, for instance. Some nights, I'll let myself indulge—I'll go out to dinner with my husband, or we'll make a buffalo chicken pizza for dinner. It's not the most calorie-friendly dinner, but the next night, I'll be sure to have something lighter. The same goes for breakfast and lunch. On Saturday morning, I might make pancakes, but on Sunday morning, I'll opt for something lighter, like an omelet or oatmeal with fruit.

I also plan most of my meals around my social life. So if I have a tasting event or party coming up, I'll watch what I eat in the days beforehand and avoid splurges like alcohol or decadent desserts, so I can enjoy them without guilt when the time arrives. It's the worst feeling when I'm at a fun event and I can't fully enjoy the experience and the goodies around me.

HOMEMADE ICED COFFEE

As you know by now, Mal and I are mad for our iced coffee. I'm sure that most of you don't need a recipe for iced coffee, but I believe my little recipe is addicting, so I've decided to add it here. The soy milk makes all the difference.

12 cups of water

8 tablespoons of ground coffee

To brew my coffee, I use a standard auto-drip coffeemaker and 12 cups of water. For 12 cups of water, I use 8 tablespoons of ground coffee. If you prefer stronger coffee, use more ground coffee (10 tablespoons); use less for weaker coffee (6 tablespoons). A good way to determine the ratio of coffee grounds to water is 1 tablespoon of coffee for every 2 cups of water. I typically use heaping spoonfuls of ground coffee because I like my iced coffee strong!

Brew coffee as you normally would; then pour it into a pitcher or thermos. If you do not have either of these, you can just put the pot itself into the fridge (let it cool a little first). Chill the iced coffee in the refrigerator overnight. Pour over ice, add a straw, and enjoy!

MAKES 12 CUPS ICED COFFEE

VANILLA CAPPUCCINO

During cold Sunday mornings when I'm looking for a hot coffee drink, I'll make this amazing vanilla cappuccino for Mal and me. The split vanilla bean makes all the difference, so don't even think of making this without it.

---

1 cup skim milk
1/2 vanilla bean, split
2 teaspoons honey
11/2 cups double-strength brewed coffee
Ground cinnamon for dusting

Put the milk and vanilla bean in a 2-cup glass measure, and microwave on high power until bubbles form around the edges, about 90 seconds. Remove the glass measure from the microwave, cover, and let steep for 5 minutes.

Scrape the vanilla seeds into the milk, and discard the pod. Stir in the honey until it is dissolved. Pour the milk into a blender, and blend until frothy, about 45 seconds.

Pour the brewed coffee into 2 mugs so they are half full, and add the milk to fill. Sprinkle with the cinnamon.

MAKES 2 DRINKS

ZUCCHINI AND TOMATO FRITTATA

Often I'll make this frittata for lunch on the weekends when I have a little extra time. It's a great way to use summer tomatoes, but it's good any time of year. Just be sure to splurge on the tomatoes. They need to be ripe and juicy.

1 tablespoon olive oil

3 medium zucchini (1 1/2 pounds), cut into 1/4-inch-thick rounds

1 small onion, finely diced

1 teaspoon dried oregano leaves, crushed

3/4 teaspoon kosher salt

3/4 teaspoon freshly ground black pepper

8 eggs

4 ounces skim-milk mozzarella cheese, diced

3 medium vine-ripened tomatoes, cored and thinly sliced crosswise

Preheat the oven to 425°F. Heat the oil over medium-high heat in a large nonstick skillet with an ovenproof handle and add the zucchini, onion, oregano, and 1/4 teaspoon each salt and pepper. Cover and cook for 7 minutes, stirring often, until the vegetables are soft. Uncover and cook for 3 minutes, until the liquid has evaporated.

Combine the eggs and remaining 1/2 teaspoon salt and pepper in a bowl, and whisk until blended. Pour the mixture over the vegetables in the skillet, and sprinkle with the mozzarella. Cook over medium-low heat for 5 minutes, until the edges are set, lifting the eggs with a spatula and tilting the pan so the uncooked eggs run under the cooked portion.

Arrange the tomatoes around the sides of the pan in a ring, and cook for 10 minutes, until the sides of the frittata are set but the center is slightly runny. Transfer to the oven, and bake for 10 minutes, until the center is set and the tomatoes are browned.

Remove the frittata from the pan and let stand for 5 minutes. Cut into 8 wedges.

MAKES 4 SERVINGS

MAL'S PANCAKES

While Mal makes these on the weekends, I often make them during the work week. I prepare the batter the night before and keep it in the refrigerator. In the morning I can have pancakes on the table in minutes.

---

1 1/2 cups all-purpose flour

   3 teaspoons baking powder

   1 teaspoon salt

   1 tablespoon sugar

1 1/2 cups vanilla soy milk

   3 ounces low-fat vanilla yogurt

   1 egg

   1 teaspoon canola oil

Combine all ingredients in a large mixing bowl. Coat a griddle (or skillet) with nonstick cooking spray, and heat the griddle until hot but not smoking over medium heat. Drop batter by the ¼ cup onto the griddle. Cook the pancakes for 2 to 3 minutes, and then flip them over. Cook the other side for about 1 minute. Serve with your favorite toppings.

MAKES 8 PANCAKES

HERBED BUTTER POPCORN

Mal and I love potato chips (who doesn't?), but now we are both enjoying this little snack as a healthier alternative. Just a touch of butter and oil really does go a long way.

- 4 cups freshly air-popped popcorn
- 1/2 teaspoon salt
- 1 tablespoon unsalted butter
- 1 tablespoon corn oil or extra-virgin olive oil
- 1/2 teaspoon cumin
- 1/4 teaspoon cayenne
- 1 tablespoon finely chopped fresh cilantro

Put the popcorn in a large bowl, and sprinkle with the salt. Toss to coat. Melt the butter in the oil in a small skillet over medium-high heat. Add the cumin and cook, stirring, until fragrant, about 30 seconds; then stir in the cayenne. Pour the mixture over the popcorn and toss to coat. Add the cilantro and toss to mix.

MAKES ABOUT 4 CUPS

13

THE MOST IMPORTANT MEAL OF THE DAY

Sometimes there's a lot of climbing on and falling off the healthy-living wagon. What can I say? I like to enjoy myself. But what keeps me moving forward when I get off track is a healthy breakfast. Starting my day with a nutritious meal always gets me back to my healthy habits.

I wake up to a grumbling stomach, which isn't unusual, considering I eat dinner so early the night before. When I was growing up, my family always ate dinner around five thirty, when my mom got home from work. I played sports in junior high and high school, so after practice or a game, I'd be famished and ready to eat dinner. Now I find that if I eat earlier in the evening, I sleep more soundly than I would with a full stomach. Plus, I really like waking up hungry for a big, hearty breakfast. It's the most important meal of the day!

A Healthy Start

My grumbling stomach immediately makes me think about what to make for breakfast, and my mind wanders from the usual bowl of oatmeal to more interesting options, like scrambled eggs with buffalo sauce or some cinnamon–brown sugar pancakes. But then thoughts of my weekend enter my head, and I remember all the high-calorie foods and cocktails I indulged in. I don't beat myself up. What's the point of getting down on myself? Plus, these weren't major slipups, so I don't need to drastically cut down on what I eat today to balance out the extra calories. Eventually, it all evens out. What I need to do is make sure to have a healthy breakfast.

I never used to eat breakfast. When I was trying to lose weight, skipping breakfast seemed like a perfectly logical way to help me cut calories and lose pounds. But I learned early on in my weight-loss efforts that this was one of the reasons I wasn't losing weight. I now know that I need to start my day with a hearty breakfast: a combination of protein, healthy fat, and fiber that will keep me full until lunchtime. If this triangle isn't complete, I inevitably end up snacking midmorning. Today, no matter how little time I have, I make sure that I throw together some sort of breakfast that will keep me going until lunch.

Eventually, I decide to make an oatmeal pancake with banana slices and peanut butter for breakfast. The combination of hearty-healthy and fiber-packed oats with protein-filled egg whites and peanut butter will stick with me all morning long. It's also a quick meal—start to finish, an oatmeal pancake probably takes 10 minutes or less to make (recipe on page 151). And, most important, a peanut butter and banana oatmeal pancake is a delicious break-fast—one of my favorite flavor combinations ever.

One Fruit, One Veg

I make sure my breakfast includes at least a serving of a fruit or vegetable every morning. Making a conscious effort to include nutritious produce starts my day off on the right foot, and it's a little reminder to live my life well beginning with my first meal of the day. Even if I don't have a lot of time for breakfast, I always manage to grab a piece of fruit. The ones with rinds are most easily transportable! My favorite grab-and-go fruits are bananas, oranges, and clementines. It's funny how such a small thing can give my whole day a new perspective.

I love nut butters, especially peanut butter, which makes it a food that is easy to go overboard with. Just recently, I realized that I finished a whole jar of peanut butter in less than one week. Apparently, I was grossly overestimating my peanut butter portion sizes. Oops! I was eating peanut butter with everything—in my oatmeal and smoothies, on toast and pita bread, and mashed up with banana. Unconsciously, I got a little out of control with the peanut butter. While it's a deliciously healthy treat, it certainly isn't low calorie.

I keep my peanut butter "problem" in mind as I begin to mix the ingredients, so I make sure to stick to my measuring spoons when it comes time to portion out the peanut butter for the top of my oatmeal pancake. The tablespoon reminds me what a serving of peanut butter looks like, which helps me cut extra calories from my breakfast without making me feel deprived. It's so easy for me to overestimate portion sizes of my favorite foods.

One Measured Tablespoon

While my pancake cooks, I make myself an iced coffee with soy milk. I'm all about multitasking! In the time that it takes me to pour the iced coffee into a glass, and add ice and soy milk, the pancake batter begins to bubble. I flip it and allow it to cook for another couple of minutes. Once the pancake is finished cooking, I place it on a plate and smear one measured tablespoon of peanut butter on top. I make sure to spread it nice and neat like a good food blogger. This meal is going to end up on my blog, so it better look appetizing!

In order to make an attractive scene for my breakfast photo shoot, I make sure to use all of the necessary food blogger elements: daylight, colorful placemats, and an appealing background. Once I have created a nice scene for my banana oatmeal pancake and iced coffee, I position them on my seasonal placemat and snap away. I start with zoomed-in shots of the edge of the pancakes, individual banana slices, and the milky iced coffee on top of the iced cubes in my glass. As soon as I have enough up-close shots, I move on to the aerial view of the entire meal. I like seeing all of the food together in one shot.

By the time I am finished with this process, my oatmeal pancake is lukewarm, which is better than cold! I'm starving, so I don't even consider reheating it. My first bite is delicious: oats, banana, and peanut butter all in one bite. In fact, it tastes so good, it's hard to believe it's a nutritious meal.

OATMEAL PANCAKE

A delicious, guilt-free pancake. (Just remember to control the amount of goodies you put on top!)

1/3 cup Quaker® Quick 1 Minute Oats

1/3 cup liquid egg whites

1/2 teaspoon baking powder

1/2 teaspoon vanilla extract

    Cinnamon

    Topping of your choice: Maple syrup, peanut butter,
      canned pumpkin, or fresh fruit

In a mixing bowl, combine the oats, egg whites, baking powder, vanilla extract, and cinnamon to taste.

Spray a 10-inch nonstick skillet with cooking spray and heat skillet over medium-low heat until hot but not smoking. Pour the batter into the pan while shaping it into a large disc with a spoon. When you can shake the pancake around in the pan it's time to flip. Cook for another few minutes until cooked through, then serve with the topping of your choice.

MAKES 1 PANCAKE

CINNAMON–BROWN SUGAR PANCAKES

The yogurt keeps these pancakes light and moist. If you have the time, slice some apples and sauté them for a few minutes in a little bit of butter; then sprinkle them with a bit of cinnamon–brown sugar. Yum.

1   cup Quaker Old Fashioned Oats

6   ounces Oikos honey yogurt

1/2 cup all-purpose flour

2   eggs

2   tablespoons canola oil

2   tablespoons brown sugar

1   teaspoon ground cinnamon

2   teaspoons vanilla extract

1   teaspoon baking powder

Combine all the ingredients in a large mixing bowl, and blend well. Spray a large nonstick skillet with vegetable oil cooking spray and heat skillet over medium-low heat until hot but not smoking.

Measure the batter in ¼-cup portions onto the pan. Cook each pancake until bubbles begin to form in the center, about 2 minutes. Flip, and cook for 2 minutes more. Serve warm.

MAKES 6 PANCAKES

BAKED BANANA OATMEAL

Unique, yes, but this is so good and so good for you. The chia seeds are the new flaxseed. They have lots of healthy omega-3s (even more than flax!), calcium, and iron, and they don't need to be ground (like flaxseeds do). Tastewise, they're sort of nutty and a little bit chewy. I use them all the time in oatmeal and smoothies.

- 1 cup Quaker Old Fashioned Oats
- 1/2 cup chopped walnuts
- 2 tablespoons brown sugar
- 1 tablespoon chia seeds (optional)
- 1/2 teaspoon baking powder
- 1/2 teaspoon ground cinnamon
- 1/4 teaspoon grated nutmeg
- 1 cup almond milk
- 1 teaspoon vanilla extract
- 1 banana

Preheat the oven to 350°F. Coat a loaf pan with nonstick cooking spray. Combine all ingredients except the banana in a mixing bowl, and pour batter into pan, spreading evenly with a spatula. Slice the banana and place it on top of the oatmeal batter. Bake for 30 minutes, or until top is lightly browned. Allow to cool before cutting.

MAKES 2 TO 4 SERVINGS

BAKED PUMPKIN OATMEAL

For a warm, sweet, cakelike oatmeal, give this instant oatmeal recipe a try!

1   packet of maple brown sugar instant oatmeal

1/4 cup canned pumpkin

1/4 cup liquid egg whites

1/2 teaspoon baking powder

Combine all ingredients in a microwave-safe bowl, and mix well. Cook in microwave on high for 2 minutes. Allow to cool before enjoying.

MAKES 1 SERVING

ALMOND BUTTER–STUFFED FRENCH TOAST

A tiny bit of almond butter makes everything taste better, and this French toast is no exception.

- 2 eggs
- 2 tablespoons milk
- 1/4 teaspoon vanilla extract
- 1/4 teaspoon ground cinnamon
- 2 tablespoons almond butter
- 4 slices thinly sliced whole wheat bread

Combine eggs, milk, vanilla, and cinnamon in a shallow bowl, and mix well. Spread almond butter on two pieces of bread (one side only) and top with the other two slices of bread to make two sandwiches. Coat both sandwiches with the egg batter. Spray a nonstick skillet with vegetable oil cooking spray and heat skillet over moderate heat until hot but not smoking. Cook the sandwiches in the skillet, 2 to 3 minutes on each side. Top the French toast with maple syrup if desired.

MAKES 2 SERVINGS

BREAKFAST RICE PUDDING

Creamy and delicious, this recipe is easy to customize, so be sure to add your favorite ingredients to the rice along with the soy milk.

---

1 cup uncooked arborio rice

1 cup vanilla soy milk

1/2 cup dried cranberries

1/2 cup almond granola

1 tablespoon brown sugar

1 teaspoon vanilla extract

Cook arborio rice as directed on the package and allow to cool in the pan for 15 to 20 minutes. Add the remaining ingredients to the rice, and stir until combined. Pour the mixture into a large plastic container, and store in the refrigerator overnight.

MAKES 4 SERVINGS

14

MURPHY, MAL, AND ME

As you've probably guessed by now, I'm just like everyone else—except that my life is all over the Internet. I had no intention of my life turning out this way, but blogging is what I love to do, and a lot of wonderful things have happened to me because of my blog.

Not every day is a wonderful, blog-tastic day. I fight with my husband, my dog destroys things, kitchen experiments blow up in my face, and technical difficulties can sometimes put me over the edge. (I've had breakdowns more than once about my blog crashing or my software not working!)

One of the areas of my life that seems pretty perfect on my blog is my relationship with my husband, Mal. And that's true: We have an amazing relationship. We laugh a lot, think the same, and rarely fight. No relationship is perfect, and there have been a number of instances over the years when things haven't turned out the way we expected, but we bend and change as needed. Our ability to adapt to new situations is one of the reasons our relationship is so strong.

My Pug Obsession

During our first year of marriage, a little pug puppy created a considerable rift in our strong relationship. Who knew that my weird pug obsession would test the strength of my marriage?

I have no idea where my obsession with pugs came from. Growing up, I actually didn't like them. My sister and I used to call the ones who lived across the street "gremlin dogs." They'd bark and snort and run around like crazy animals. They were not cute and cuddly dogs. I think we were probably scared of them, too. Some pugs are really ugly.

My family owned cats, so I never really considered myself a "dog person" until after graduating college. A co-worker of mine lived nearby and often asked me to dog-sit his pug, Curtis. I lived a thirty-second walk from his apartment, so it was easy for me to pop by and take his dog for a walk. I wasn't necessarily a fan of pugs right off the bat, but as the months passed, I got to know Curtis and his personality better. I ended up moving to a different part of the city about a year later, but for some reason, the memories of Curtis spurred my love (and eventually my obsession) for pugs.

For the next five years or so, all I did was talk about owning a pug. Unfortunately, it was never the right time to own a dog—I didn't have enough time to devote to a pet or my living situation didn't allow for a dog. Eventually, I felt like I couldn't live without a pug in my life, and I convinced Mal that we needed to get one.

Mal wasn't 100 percent on board with getting a dog. He wanted to have one in his life, but at the time, our apartment building didn't allow pets, so getting a dog meant that we would have to move. After a lot of convincing conversations, eventually he gave in and let me get the pug of my dreams.

Murphy, Mr. Personality

I researched pug breeders in the New England area on the Internet for weeks and weeks before choosing one in western Massachusetts. One afternoon in August 2009, Mal and I drove out to Sturbridge, Massachusetts, and met Murphy for the first time. From the moment I set eyes on him, I knew that he was the pug for me. He had so much personality, and he was easily the most adorable pug I had ever seen. I knew that we needed to be together. Murphy was too young for us to take home that day—and we still needed to find a new place to live—so he remained with the breeder until we figured out the next step. (Looking back, I realize that I was crazy for uprooting our simple life for a dog, but it was all worth it in the end.)

The next couple of weeks were a blur. Mal and I frantically looked for a place to live. We searched Craigslist for apartment listings and contacted Realtor after Realtor. At the time, I was working in Cambridge, so I wanted to move somewhere closer to work. (My commute was terrible!) We focused our apartment search on South Boston, which was located smack in the middle between Mal's school and my office.

At the time, South Boston made perfect sense. It's an expensive area to live because of its close proximity to the city, but I was essentially making two full-time incomes. Financially, we could afford a bigger place that was closer to the city and that allowed dogs. Mal and I were in such a rush to find a place, we snapped up the first decent one that we found: a modern, loft-style apartment in the heart of Southie. It even had a washer and dryer! But we were in such a rush to find a dog-friendly apartment, we didn't think through the negatives of the area and the apartment.

Unhappy Campers

When I look back on our move to South Boston, the whole thing seems cursed. Nothing went well when we lived there. Mal and I were both unhappy, but we decided to make the best of it and tough it out. We thought that it had to get better, but we soon realized that living in Southie would never get better. We battled with a lack of parking, snow bans (when the city forbids parking on the street so snowplows can keep the roads clear—it's a real pain in the butt, as you can imagine; there's no place to put your car!), garbage, people who didn't pick up after their dogs, and a crazy downstairs neighbor who would scream (and sometimes cry) every time she saw Murphy. South Boston just wasn't for us.

Eventually, Mal, Murphy, and I moved to a new apartment in a different area right outside Boston that fits us much better. We're much happier, and Murphy has plenty of room to stretch his pug legs. I'm so relieved that my guys are in a much more positive situation—after all, the whole Southie debacle was my idea.

Despite the moving fiasco, I am so glad that I have Murphy in my life. (Mal has come around and is now just as obsessed with Murphy as I am!) Murphy makes me happy each and every day, and I credit him with saving me from another cold, dark Boston winter of depression and sadness.

Murphy to the Rescue

During the winter, I would often find myself really down in the dumps for many weeks. Last year, I felt so lethargic and blah that I started to bail on plans with friends and even my husband, which was totally unlike me. I knew something wasn't right, but I couldn't figure it out. I tried hosting a yoga challenge on my blog to help get me out of my funk. Practicing yoga almost every day made me feel a little bit better, but I still wasn't my normal self. Eventually, I became concerned that my down-in-the-dumps mood was something more serious, so I consulted my doctor toward the end of the winter. She told me that the short days were likely affecting my mood and suspected that I had seasonal affective disorder (SAD). (Say what? I had never heard of such a thing.)

She suggested that I buy a light box, which has been proven as an effective treatment for SAD. Since it was the end of the winter, I didn't purchase a light box right away, but I knew that I needed to buy one to get me through this winter. My poor husband had to deal with my mopey moods.

Finally, I did some research and purchased a Day-Light Lamp. The light source is delivered at an angle that mimics outdoor light, so I also thought it might be good for my food photography. I used the lamp for twenty minutes a day for three or four days in a row. I didn't feel any different, but you're supposed to use the light consistently for a lot longer. I ended up getting really busy and forgetting to use it altogether, but I didn't get the "winter blues" like I had year after year.

Turns out that my little pug creature saved me from SAD this year. Seriously, I laugh at Murphy every single day. He makes me happy from the time I wake up until the time I fall asleep (listening to him snore like a chainsaw). I also take him for a lot of walks outside, so I get quite a bit more sunlight in my life than I did in previous years. I realize that not everyone can (or wants to) own a dog, but Murphy, for me and Mal, is pretty perfect.

VANILLA MINI CUPCAKES

Okay, I know you are not supposed to feed your dog "people food," but just occasionally Murphy and I share one of these little cupcakes, without any frosting, of course (dogs are not supposed to eat chocolate).

1/2 cup (1 stick) unsalted butter, softened

1 cup sugar

3 eggs, separated

1/2 teaspoon vanilla extract

1 cup all-purpose flour

1/2 teaspoon baking powder

1/4 teaspoon baking soda

1/8 teaspoon salt

1/2 cup buttermilk

Prepared frosting (optional)

Preheat the oven to 350°F and grease 24 mini-muffin cups with butter. Combine the butter and sugar in a large bowl, and beat with an electric mixer at high speed until light and fluffy. Beat in the egg yolks and vanilla, and set aside. Clean and dry the beaters.

Combine the flour, baking powder, baking soda, and salt in a sifter, and sift onto waxed paper. Beat the egg whites in a bowl with the mixer at high speed until soft peaks form when the beaters are raised.

CONTINUED

Add one-fourth of the flour mixture to the butter mixture, alternately with one-third of the buttermilk, beginning and ending with the flour mixture (do not overbeat). Fold in the egg whites using a plastic spatula.

Spoon the batter into the prepared cups. Bake until the tops of the cakes spring back when lightly pressed with your finger, 15 to 20 minutes. Cool the cakes in the pans on a wire rack for 5 minutes. Remove from the pans and cool completely. Frost as desired.

MAKES 24 MINI CUPCAKES

15

GETTING OFF THE COUCH

I have always been an active person. As a toddler, I began dancing—ballet, tap, and jazz—and by the time I was eight years old, I played soccer every spring and fall until college. In high school, I really started to get into fitness. Besides soccer, I ran track, played tennis, skied, and took group exercise classes at the local health club. My love for exercise continued into college, when I started running a few times a week. It wasn't until I started working full-time that I struggled to find time to exercise.

In the summer of 2009, I had the opportunity to talk to Bob Greene, Oprah Winfrey's friend and fitness guru. He was hosting a conference call with a group of health-minded bloggers, and I was asked if I wanted to participate. Of course, I accepted this wonderful opportunity to chat with such a motivational individual.

When it was time for the call, I dialed in, introduced myself to the group, and waited patiently to speak with Bob Greene himself. My brain was on overdrive thinking about what I should say. Soon, Bob introduced himself to the group, and each blogger had a moment to introduce him- or herself and say hello to Bob. I was incredibly nervous, but I was able to briefly introduce myself and my blog.

The rest of the call was a roundtable conversation, and each participant could ask Bob a question about anything. I didn't want to waste my opportunity; I wanted to ask a question that I hoped would have a really useful answer. Recently, my life had become very hectic: I had a full-time job in addition to the blog and my freelance writing, I was planning a healthy-living conference, and I had a new puppy. Exercise was the first thing to go from my daily routine. So I asked Bob how I could squeeze more exercise into my life.

Bob's response actually caught me by surprise. He said that I needed to change my perspective about exercise. Bob explained that exercise shouldn't be something that I squeeze into my life. Instead it should be a priority in my life—something that I do every day, almost like brushing my teeth. Fitness should be something that I make time for no matter what. Being fit is necessary for a happy and healthy life, so why not make it an important element of my lifestyle? As soon as he said this, a light bulb went off in my head. It was definitely an aha moment for me!

From that day forward, I made fitness a priority in my life. I planned my exercise for the day and then fit all the other elements around it. When I changed my perspective about fitness, it helped me reprioritize what is most important to me with regard to my health—and it has also made "fitting" fitness in my life so much easier. I would rarely go more than a day or two without incorporating some sort of activity in my day. Exercise became essential "me time," a reward for all the hard work I do in other areas of my life. A sweaty workout would always seem to melt away the stress.

Sounds great, right? Unfortunately, this fairy tale didn't last forever. About six months after I spoke with Bob Greene, my motivation for fitness really started to wane. I was back to my old ways, trying to "squeeze" exercise into my life, and not really pushing myself at the gym. I'd spend thirty minutes on the elliptical, not break a sweat, and call it a day. Plus, I barely made time for strength training. I'd halfheartedly do a set or two of upper-body strength training, but I wouldn't work my muscles to fatigue and I'd wake up the next morning feeling like I hadn't worked out at all. Soon, my arms and legs started to get a little flabby. The muscle definition that I loved seeing was nowhere to be found, and I started to feel really bad about myself.

I really hate it when people complain about their lives and do nothing to change them. What's the point in being unhappy if you can do something to change your situation and make it better? Without realizing it, I became one of these people.

One night, after dinner, Mal and I were relaxing and watching TV. We had just finished dinner and I was feeling a bit depressed. I had overeaten, so my stomach was uncomfortably full and my body just felt gross from skipping the gym one too many days in a row. I was cranky and disappointed in how I was treating my body—and I started to complain. Like the nice guy that he is, Mal listened for a few minutes, but then he turned to me and said, "Well, if you're not happy, do something about it." He was mocking me, but he was right! I say this all the time—to him, family members, friends, and even my blog readers. Of course, I mean it in the nicest way possible, but if you're not happy, do something to change it!

At that very moment, I got my lazy butt off the couch and created a plan of action. My thirtieth birthday was coming up in about six months, so I figured this occasion would be the perfect one to motivate me to "lose the dough" and shape up for good. Some people bug out about turning thirty, but I'm really looking forward to it. Entering a new decade is sort of like turning over a new leaf. It was time for me to map out my plan of attack.

I wanted to enter my thirties as my healthiest self and looking my best, so I embarked on a six-month journey to get myself in tip-top shape. I named my challenge Lose the Dough for the Big 3-0. It was a little corny, but it described my situation pretty well. It's not like I needed to lose a lot of weight, but since our wedding well over a year ago, I'd put on a few pounds—nothing major, but I still felt a little doughy. I was ripped on the day that I got married! I had big, scary muscles that I loved to show off. I worked hard for that body, but slowly and surely, the postwedding pounds caught up with me. I wanted to lose the dough for one of the most important birthdays of my lifetime.

I'm a big fan of planning and recording my workouts each week. It keeps me on track and motivated. Spending some time on Sunday night organizing my to-dos for the week allows me to figure out when I can schedule my workouts. Seeing my week laid out and organized with plenty of time for exercise motivates me to stick to my plan. Plus, there's nothing more satisfying than checking a workout off a to-do list! Keeping track of my workouts also helps me identify what works and what doesn't work in my exercise routines. For instance, every other week or so, I will go back through my recorded workouts and assess what I have been doing. Instead of just going through the motions, I look for holes in my workouts and try to switch things up.

I recently started to bake a small batch of Workout Cookies on Sunday night to motivate me to get out of bed for my workweek trips to the gym. I know you're not supposed to bribe yourself with food—especially if you're trying to lose weight—but for just 80 calories, a Workout Cookie fuels me with lots of whole grains, fiber, low-fat protein, healthy omegas, and some subtle sweetness. Just the thought of a delicious baked treat gets me out of bed—even in the cold, dark winter mornings in Boston. Plus, I usually end up burning way more than 80 calories at the gym.

But first, these are the workouts I developed as part of the Lose the Dough challenge. I tried to step up my workouts with a combination of strength training and cardio on the same day.

ANOTHER 45-MINUTE FULL-BODY STRENGTH-TRAINING WORKOUT

Seated Leg Press: 15 reps, 3 sets, 110 pounds

Single Seated Leg Press: 15 reps, 3 sets, 20 pounds

Leg Extension: 10 reps, 3 sets, 70 pounds

Hamstring Curl: 10 reps, 3 sets, 40 pounds

Chest Press: 15 reps, 3 sets, 45-pound bar

Biceps Curl to Military Press (compound exercise):
15 reps, 3 sets, 10 pounds

**Bent-over Row to Triceps Kickback
(compound exercise):** 15 reps, 3 sets, 8 pounds

Assisted Pulls: 10 reps, 2 sets (my arms were jelly!),
65 pounds

THE PYRAMID

A 25-minute treadmill walking workout.

0:00—1:00 at 4.1 mph (1.0 incline)

1:00—3:00 at 4.2 mph (2.0 incline)

3:00—6:00 at 4.3 mph (3.0 incline)

6:00—10:00 at 4.4 mph (4.0 incline)

10:00—15:00 at 4.5 mph (5.0 incline)

15:00—19:00 at 4.4 mph (4.0 incline)

19:00—22:00 at 4.3 mph (3.0 incline)

22:00—24:00 at 4.2 mph (2.0 incline)

24:00—25:00 at 4.1 mph (1.0 incline)

Variations:

Running option: Add 2.0 mph to each interval

50-minute option: Repeat workout twice.

WORKOUT COOKIES

These cookies are the perfect fuel before a workout. They provide healthy carbohydrates with a little bit of low-fat protein for staying power. They're also delicious—almost like eating a regular cookie!

- 1/4 cup whole wheat flour
- 3/4 cup Quaker Old Fashioned Oats
- 1/4 cup ground flaxseed meal
- 1/4 cup brown sugar
- 1/4 cup raisins
- 1/2 teaspoon ground cinnamon
- 6 ounces plain Greek yogurt
- 1/8 cup canola oil

Preheat the oven to 375°F. Coat a 12-cup muffin pan with nonstick cooking spray.

In a large bowl, combine all the ingredients and mix well.

Divide the batter evenly among the muffin cups (they will be only about 1/3 full). Bake for 12 to 15 minutes, or until golden brown.

MAKES 12 COOKIES

BLUEBERRY SMOOTHIE

Blueberries are considered a superfood, and I try to sprinkle them liberally over everything. Since I can get them frozen year-round, I also make this smoothie at least once a week. It is superdelicious!

1 cup frozen blueberries

1 ripe banana

1 cup nonfat plain yogurt

Combine all the ingredients in a blender, and blend on high speed until smooth.

MAKES 2 SMOOTHIES

WATERMELON QUENCHER

During the summer months, I make this whenever I can. It's ideal after a tough workout because it really does quench your thirst.

5 cups watermelon, seeds removed

2 tablespoons or more fresh lime or lemon juice

Combine the watermelon and 2 tablespoons lime or lemon juice in a blender and puree. Taste, adjust the citrus juice if desired, and blend again. Pour the liquid through a strainer into a large pitcher and drain without pressing on the solids. Skim off foam from the watermelon juice and serve over ice in tall glasses.

MAKES 2 TO 4 SERVINGS

16

. . . AND THE REST WILL FOLLOW

As I already mentioned, my love affair with health clubs started a long time ago. I joined my first gym when I was sixteen years old. I had a part-time job as a cashier at a local grocery store, and my paycheck went for the membership. I absolutely loved going to the gym. It felt like a mini-vacation or trip to the spa, with its heated pool, sauna, steam room, and hot tub. I'd spend hours there after my workout enjoying all of its finest comforts.

Of course, I loved exercising, too. At the time, in the mid- to late 1990s, step aerobics was all the rage and, like everyone else, I couldn't get enough. I'd even take two classes in one day, if I had the time. Stepping up and down and bouncing all around was such a blast for me. Plus, I was getting my heart pumping and burning some calories. Since I had been taking dance lessons from the time I was a toddler, no choreography was too difficult—the more intricate the combination, the better. I was always the first person to "get it" in the class. While the instructor spent a good five minutes showing the rest of the class how to do a new move, I had it mastered after the first time I saw it. Before I knew it, my classmates would start placing their steps around mine just so they could follow along with what I was doing.

Despite having confidence in my step aerobics skills, I never liked to show them off. I always put myself in the back right-hand corner of the room. It was weird and uncomfortable for other people in the class to watch my every move. I liked helping people, but having a half dozen people stare at me bugged me out.

You Have to Laugh

I have a lot more confidence today than I did back then, but there are still many times when I feel self-conscious at the gym, although for entirely different reasons. One morning in the dead of winter, I put on my workout gear in my cold, dark bedroom and headed straight to the gym. When I got there, I hopped on the elliptical and started peddling away like most mornings—until I looked down and noticed my sneaker—my purple-and-gray sneaker, from the pair that I wore only when doing yard work or tromping through the woods. That's when I realized that my sneakers didn't match. I had on one purple sneaker and one white sneaker. At first, I didn't really care—and who would notice? The important thing was that I made it to the gym and was exercising. Not five minutes later, one of the trainers walked by me and said, "Nice sneakers, Punky Brewster." Of course, he said it loud enough for everyone around me to hear. Apparently, someone did notice my mismatching sneakers, and now everyone else in the cardio section would notice too. I must have looked like such a nerd. I ended up cutting my workout short that morning.

Luxury Helps

Even so, I love my gym. It's an upscale all-women's gym called Healthworks in downtown Boston. It has six locations in and around the city, and it is easily the best women's gym in the area. It has the best classes, most knowledgeable fitness staff, and programming and events that change every month. There's always something new to try out or get involved with. And the location where I work out most has a full-service spa, where you can treat yourself to some rest and relaxation after working hard at the gym.

The facilities are gorgeous, and the equipment is brand-new—even the bath products in the locker room are nice! I've been known to spend half a day there—taking an hour-long class, dillydallying in the sauna and then the shower, and treating myself to a facial before I head home. It's like a mini-vacation or a day at the spa. It's quality alone time with myself to just relax and unwind. Plus, it's a nice way to get in a workout!

Healthworks is also infamous for its outrageous monthly dues. While it's the best women's gym in the Boston area, it's also the most expensive. But you get what you pay for, and for me, paying exorbitant fees is an investment in my health. And since I hate wasting money, just the thought of blowing a hundred dollars each month gets my butt to the gym—and isn't that the most important thing?

Finding My Way

Exercising and spending time at Healthworks actually inspired me to pursue a career change to become a personal trainer. For four months in the fall of 2008, I worked as a fitness specialist in the evenings after my full-time job. My position included answering questions from members, providing fitness assessments, and giving orientations to free weights and the Nautilus machines. Meanwhile, I studied to become a certified personal trainer using an at-home study course that would prepare me to take a computerized exam in a few months. Once I was certified, my plan was to quit my full-time job and become a personal trainer at Healthworks. But after a few months of working a full-time job, working a part-time job, blogging, and trying to study for the certification exam, I had a mini–mental breakdown. The stress was too much, and I couldn't handle it. The combination of responsibilities and expectations that I had for myself was too overwhelming. I had bitten off much more than I could chew, and I needed to reassess.

After a good, long crying session, I realized what I wanted to do—and being a personal trainer was not it.

Selling myself to get clients didn't fit my personality. After some serious soul-searching, I decided that a career change was much too drastic for me, and a life devoted to health and wellness did not necessarily mean that it also had to be my full-time job. (Oh, how wrong I was about this!)

At the Harvard School of Public Health (HSPH), I was the program coordinator for the masters of public health (MPH) program. It was a small office with just four people, so I got to be involved with a lot of aspects of the program. My main responsibilities were managing the MPH Web site, organizing MPH-sponsored events like lectures and seminars, counseling students on their degree require-ments, keeping track of curriculum changes and notifying students, coordinating the logistics for the summer session, taking minutes at MPH steering committee meetings, and gathering students' culminating experience reports (their master's theses). I stayed for more than three years. The pace of the office was pretty slow, so I had time to write the blog during work hours. (Don't tell my boss!) I actually had time to put some thought into my posts and post three times a day, which likely helped grow my readership in the beginning. I also had time to comment on other people's blogs, which helped market mine even more because readers would click through to *Carrots 'N' Cake.*

I then moved on to become the executive assistant to the dean of Harvard College. I left HSPH to find a position that was more "exciting," figuring that if I had a full-time job that I really loved, maybe I'd forget about my dream of blogging full-time. My husband and I must have had fifty conversations about the future of *Carrots 'N' Cake.* I was making money through an advertiser, but not nearly enough to live off of. Basically, blogging full-time was a big dream.

I started at Harvard College in January 2009 with high hopes for a new life. I thought working in the middle of the action at Harvard, being the right-hand assistant to the dean, would fulfill me, but within just a few months I knew that it wasn't the job for me. My main role was managing the dean's calendar. I love organization, so at first I thought it was "fun" to arrange meetings and maximize the dean's time to the best of my ability. Scheduling meetings and making sure they all jived together was a challenge that I enjoyed. But it got old real quick. I knew that I couldn't do the job forever.

Overwhelmed, Sound Familiar?

That spring, I secured a freelance writing job with Health. com. My gig with Health was 100 percent luck and good timing! I e-mailed Health to inquire about some freelance work and, at the same time, they were looking for someone who had lost weight and maintained it to contribute to their Feel Great Weight program. A few of the Health editors were readers of my blog, so that helped too. This writing job provided me with an additional income, but it still wasn't quite enough to live on, especially in an expensive city like Boston.

One of the biggest sources of my stress was being totally overwhelmed by my lack of a work–life balance. I was working a full-time job, blogging, and freelance writing. Even when I was sleeping, my brain was still thinking about work. I dreaded Monday mornings so much that on Sunday nights, I was practically sick with anxiety about the upcoming workweek. To me, life is just way too short to be miserable at your job. You spend the majority of your day working it, so if you are absolutely hating it, you hate most days. This is not a great mentality to have. Something had to go.

I had considered devoting less time to my blog, but I'm not the type of person who can do something halfway, especially a project that I have already devoted so much time and energy to. My blog is my baby! In the end, I decided that giving up *Carrots 'N' Cake* was just not an option, but how the heck would I pay the bills if I resigned from my full-time job to devote more time to it?

Sleepless in Boston

During the spring and summer of that year, Mal and I had a bunch of heart-to-heart talks that would almost always end with me in tears. I didn't have enough time for the blog, but I knew I couldn't give up on my dream that easily. Plus, I was miserable dealing with an hour commute each way to my full-time job and trying to keep up with my blog, freelance work, and everything else. Of course, I couldn't really talk about my situation much on the blog for privacy reasons (and because my boss and co-workers read it), but the late summer and early fall of 2009 was a very low time in my life. I kept the positive image and smile on my face, but some nights, the stress would be so overwhelming that I would cry myself to sleep. Some nights, I wouldn't even sleep at all because there was so much on my mind. I dreaded going to work every day. My heart was somewhere else, and, in short, I was a miserable person.

You know when you get that feeling in the pit of your stomach that you have to do something and there's no other way? That was the way I felt. I couldn't live my life being miserable at work, and I knew what I had to do. I needed to figure out a roadmap to my ultimate goal and then get behind the wheel and drive. I knew it might not happen right away or even in the next few months (or even a year), but I knew that if I wanted it bad enough, it would happen. It all started with a choice.

Holdin' On

And then *Carrots 'N' Cake* started to take off. All sorts of opportunities started to present themselves, and I was receiving positive feedback from my readers. I was inspired. Looking back, I now see that my blog got me through one of the hardest times of my life. After a crappy day at work, I could write out my thoughts and start to feel a bit better about things. I loved reading comments and answering questions from readers. It made me feel good to help people.

I'm pretty straight and narrow when it comes to job security and a steady paycheck, so I knew quitting my job and hoping that my *Carrots 'N' Cake* income would get me by was a bad idea. As much as I wanted to impulsively quit my full-time job and devote all my time to blogging, I took the time to make a calculated decision in order to make my dream a reality without totally messing up my life.

While working at Harvard, I was planning behind the scenes. I started by creating a list of what I thought would make me happy; then I considered all of the possible ways to make that happen. I consulted my husband a lot during this time. Ultimately, the decision was all mine, but almost daily, I bounced ideas off him. Mal brought me back to reality and prevented me from rushing into anything (which is sometimes what I do). At the same time, he supported and encouraged me to chase my dream.

Taking Steps

After weeks of considering possible options, I finally formulated a plan of attack: save money (for when I leave my full-time job); research part-time jobs related to health, wellness, nutrition, and the like; secure a part-time job (that will pay the bills); resign from my current job to devote more time to blogging; try not to freak out; seek out additional social media projects for extra income. And, that's just what I did . . . minus the not-freaking-out part. I did plenty of that!

Once I formulated my plan of attack, I went into supersave mode and cut back on everything. I didn't go out to eat, didn't buy clothing, didn't buy any extras. I opened a high-interest savings account and saved about half of my income. I squirreled away every little bit that I could and was able to save a good chunk of my income as a security blanket for when I finally resigned from my full-time job. It was the best thing I ever did.

And I spent a lot of time looking for part-time jobs. I wasn't going to leave my fancy-schmancy Harvard job for any old gig, I wanted a job that was related to my passions and that would allow me some flexibility in my schedule. I applied for quite a few jobs and went on a number of interviews. A few months later, I finally got the call I had been waiting for—I was offered a part-time job working for a company that I truly believe in. The new position was working for a nutritional rating company called NuVal, and I'd be in charge of their social media. It was the perfect job for me—it related to my health and wellness passions and it was very much in line with my career goals. In October 2009, I resigned from my full-time job at Harvard.

So how did my dream job come about? A few months before, NuVal's mommy blogger contacted me about doing a guest post on *Carrots 'N' Cake*. At first, I almost deleted her e-mail. I get requests like this all of the time from random people who just want to use my blog as a vehicle to get their company's name out into the blog world. But I noticed that the company was located right outside Boston, so I visited the NuVal website and did some research. NuVal is a scientifically based nutritional scoring system that rates foods on how nutritious they are on a scale of 1 to 100. Consumers use the scoring system across all products and brands to make informed decisions about food. It was a perfect match with my interest in nutrition and wellness!

One important thing I have learned in life is that if you want something, *ask for it*! You might as well try to get what you want. I mean, the worst-case scenario is that you get a "no," right? So I asked if NuVal was looking to hire anyone. I knew that I wanted to be involved with this company in some capacity, but what did I want to do? Eventually the folks at NuVal invited me in for an "exploratory" conversation. We chatted about their goals and future plans, and then we discussed how I could benefit the company. I put on my game face and pitched myself: I wanted to do social media marketing for them.

I left the meeting feeling pretty confident, but a few weeks later, I still hadn't heard anything. So what did I do? I followed up like a crazy person! I sent examples of my writing, videos about the benefits of social media—I even sent a sample job description. I was probably on the verge of being annoying, but I knew this potential job opportunity would be the perfect fit for me. I just couldn't let it slip away! To make a long story short, I got the job! My new workweek is divided between my blogging career and my new role as a social media strategist. With my obvious interest in nutrition and social media, NuVal seems like the perfect fit for me.

Although I may not make as much money as I used to, I wake up every morning excited about the day. When I started my blog, I knew it would help me keep on track with my healthy habits. And while my new healthy lifestyle eventually changed many different aspects of my life, I never guessed that it would score me a new job!

Needless to say, after getting the job, I decided to celebrate with my favorite pumpkin muffins.

PUMPKIN CAROB CHIP MUFFINS

There are so many good things in these muffins that you can feel pretty virtuous having one of them. And if you make mini-muffins, you'll be saving even more calories.

1 cup plain canned pumpkin

1/3 cup water

1/3 cup canola oil

2 tablespoons ground flaxseeds

1 teaspoon vanilla

12/3 cups whole wheat flour

11/3 cups sugar

1 teaspoon baking powder

1/2 teaspoon baking soda

1/2 teaspoon kosher salt

1/2 teaspoon ground cinnamon

1/4 teaspoon grated nutmeg

2/3 cup vegan carob chips

Preheat the oven to 350°F. Spray a nonstick muffin tin with nonstick cooking spray or line the tin with paper muffin cups and spray the cups with nonstick cooking spray.

Put the pumpkin, water, canola oil, ground flaxseeds, and vanilla in a blender, and process on high for at least 1 minute, until light in color and well blended.

Whisk together the whole wheat flour, sugar, baking powder, baking soda, salt, cinnamon, and nutmeg in a large mixing bowl. Add the pumpkin mixture, and mix well with a wooden spoon or large spatula until well blended. Fold in the carob chips.

Spoon the batter into the muffin tin, distributing evenly. Bake for 10 to 12 minutes, until a wooden pick (or knife) inserted near the center comes out clean. Let the muffins cool for 5 minutes in the pan, then use a spatula to gently lift each muffin from the tin. Finish cooling on a wire rack.

MAKES 12 MUFFINS OR ABOUT 26 MINI-MUFFINS

OATMEAL RAISIN BARS

Sometimes it is easier to make a pan of bars than a batch of cookies.
If you are an oatmeal cookie person like me, these are a must.

2 cups old-fashioned oats

1 cup raisins

3/4 cup all-purpose flour

1/2 cup packed brown sugar

1/2 cup canola oil

2 eggs

1/2 teaspoon ground cinnamon

1/4 teaspoon salt

Preheat the oven to 350°F, and spray an 8- by 8-inch baking pan with nonstick cooking spray. Combine all the ingredients in a large mixing bowl until smooth. Spread the batter in the baking pan, and bake for 25 to 30 minutes, until a wooden pick (or knife) inserted near the center comes out clean. Let the bars cool completely before cutting.

MAKES 9 BARS

17

TRAVEL
EATS

When Mal and I took a trip to the West Coast last year, I did my best to not let my healthy eating habits take a vacation too. Maintaining my weight loss is a whole different story when I go on vacation. Still, with not a lot of effort, I was able to incorporate a number of (painless) healthy strategies into my trip.

When I used to travel before losing weight, my bad habits began before I even left the airport. In fact, while waiting for my flight, I sought out a humongous chocolate chip muffin—what better time to splurge than vacation, right? I hated the challenge of maintaining a diet while I was supposed to be relaxing. But

I've learned that if I want to continue to fit into my jeans, a little motivation and planning go a long way.

Jeans vs. Baggy Pants

These days, I feel it's important to maintain healthy eating even on vacation. If I indulge too much, I feel a little bit guilty. But, at the same time, it's *vacation*: I should be able to splurge, so I allow myself to do so at most meals. I just do my best to balance the healthy with the not-so-healthy. So, for instance, I might eat a light breakfast to save room for a splurge at lunch, or I'll go for a run first thing in the morning, so I can splurge at breakfast with a mimosa or chocolate chip muffin. Typically, I won't overdo snacks on vacations because I know my meals will be pretty indulgent. Plus, eating bigger meals usually holds off my hunger. It's not that I would gain very much weight in a single week; I just don't like feeling that I did. If I overeat, I feel blah about myself. I like coming back from vacation feeling rejuvenated, which, for me, means healthy.

I used to stick to baggy sweats for long plane rides. Of course, I was comfortable, but this type of clothing made me so relaxed that I forgot all about my healthy habits. And since I could barely see my body, I had no problem snacking throughout the whole flight—usually on low-quality, high-calorie plane food. Now when I travel, I make sure to wear formfitting, stylish clothing that makes me feel confident about myself. For me, wearing an attractive outfit is a constant reminder to stay on track with my healthy habits. Plus, it's not comfortable to overeat when I am wearing tight jeans!

I also used to think that people who brought their own food on vacation were uptight control freaks, but I've learned that with a little advance planning, eating on the road doesn't have to be a burden. It is vacation, after all, so I'll splurge on something fun at the airport, like a soy milk Misto to pair with a Lärabar or homemade peanut butter and jelly on whole wheat bread. And since I sometimes confuse thirst for hunger, I bring a big bottle of water and stay away from sodas and alcohol. If I'm taking a road trip, I always make sure to store a cooler in the backseat with pre-made sandwiches, yogurt, low-fat cheese, and whole-grain crackers or fresh fruit.

I also pack a couple of emergency snacks for my trips. In the past, I've gotten myself in a lot of trouble by waiting until I was in the middle of a desperate hunger situation. I'd spend the afternoon sightseeing and then, starving, I'd come across a fast-food restaurant that didn't offer many healthy options, and suddenly a large chocolate milk shake sounded really appealing! So if I know that I have a full day ahead of me, I make sure to pack nutritious snacks to control my hunger. And if I have to settle for something that's not on my healthy list, I remember that I can still control the size of the portion.

Instead of obsessing over the food, I focus my attention on my entire vacation experience, including the sights, sounds, and people on my trip. And instead of spending money on overpriced, high-calorie foods, I save my dollars for nonedible souvenirs and beauty treats (hello, rejuvenating massage!).

I never used to exercise on vacation. Vacation was supposed to mean a break from my normal routine. I'd spend my time lounging around, sipping cocktails, and munching on less-than-nutritious snacks, which left me feeling sluggish and unhappy with myself. Now I try to include some sort of exercise on all of my vacations to keep myself feeling confident. I've learned that not everyone on my vacation enjoys planning active things like walking tours, hiking, and running though a new city—but I still make exercise a priority for me. On my various trips, I've packed resistance bands and exercise DVDs, and I've used the television guide to find exercise programs that allow me to work out in the comfort of my hotel room. I also make sure to pack my sneakers and iPod for a quick jog to offset some of those extra vacation calories. I like to run first thing in the morning before everyone else wakes up so I don't miss out on the activities planned for later in the day. If I can't find time for a workout, even a brisk walk after dinner makes me feel good and helps me stick to my healthy habits.

Plan the Splurge

Now when I splurge on a vacation meal, not just any food will do—it has to be worth it! When we visited Victoria, British Columbia, Mal and I planned a special wine tour and three-course lunch. Calorie-wise, the wine tour and lunch were a big splurge, but it was a conscious overindulgence with lasting memories—instead of just regular old vacation fare that didn't mean much. To balance out the extra calories, I planned to eat a light breakfast and dinner, so I could fully enjoy my special wine tour with my hubby.

When dining out on vacation, I would have helped myself to the bread basket, enjoyed a glass of wine, and ordered an appetizer, an entrée, and dessert at a restaurant. I wanted to try everything and didn't pay attention to portion sizes. Rather than repress my foodie urges, I learned to trim my portion sizes up front. On our recent vacation, my husband and I dined at a Spanish tapas restaurant. Tapas are a great way to taste a number of different dishes but avoid the inflated portion sizes. By ordering less, I didn't overindulge and, at the same time, it adjusted my image of how much to eat. If "small plates" aren't an option, I pair an appetizer with a salad or soup for my meal, which allows me to enjoy many foods of smaller portion sizes.

Think Options

The hotel where we stayed offered a free continental breakfast. Back before I paid attention to what I ate, I would have picked a fruit Danish and a cup of coffee. A sugary pastry inevitably set me up for disaster because it lacked staying power—I'd be hungry just a couple of hours later. Now I know the importance of incorporating protein and some healthy fats into my breakfast. If the continental breakfast has a hot bar, I order scrambled eggs or an egg-white omelet. If my breakfast options are limited, yogurt with cereal or an English muffin with peanut butter and fresh fruit are my go-to foods. If the only choices at the continental breakfast are enormous bagels and donuts, I seek out my own healthy foods at a local farmers' market or grocery store, which are typically easy to find and provide a unique opportunity to explore the area and try new items.

While on vacation, Mal and I often decide to eat a few meals in, saving both money and calories. For breakfast, it's easy to pack some tried-and-true foods, like instant oatmeal and Lärabars. Eating in for lunch and dinner are great opportunities to include high-nutrient, high-fiber fruits and vegetables. Veggie-packed sandwiches and salads, for example, are easy ways to get your vegetables, and they don't require much prep work. Typically, a market or grocery store with lots of good-for-you options is just a few minutes away and almost as easy as ordering a meal from a restaurant. We use the money we save to order a special glass of wine or buy an extra souvenir from our trip.

It's easy to overdo it when surrounded by new and delicious foods on vacation. I stick to a few healthy strategies during my trip, and when I return, I make sure that my very first meal at home is packed with whole foods, and then I move on.

I used to get really upset when my clothing would be tight after a vacation or indulgent holiday, but all of that worrying and disappointment never did me any good. Instead I changed my thinking: gaining weight is a "problem" that can be fixed. So I thought back to how I felt when I first began losing weight, and I remembered the excitement and the high expectations of weight loss. Rekindling these feelings instantly motivated me to work hard toward my goal once again.

SPICED PECANS

Whenever I travel by car, I try to tote along a plastic bag filled with these nuts . . . so good, but remember, just a few at a time!

1   tablespoon canola or grapeseed oil

4   teaspoons Worcestershire sauce

2   teaspoons ground cumin

2   teaspoons ground coriander

1   teaspoon chili powder

1   teaspoon fine sea salt

1/8 teaspoon cayenne

1   pound pecan halves

Preheat the oven to 300°F. Line a baking sheet with parchment paper. Combine the oil, Worcestershire sauce, cumin, coriander, chili powder, salt, and cayenne in a medium bowl, and mix until blended. Add the pecans, and toss well to coat.

Spread the pecans on the prepared baking sheet, and bake until crisp and fragrant, about 20 minutes, stirring after 10 minutes. Let cool completely; then store in jars.

MAKES 4 CUPS

BROWNIES WITH A SECRET

*Prune puree makes these brownies extra rich without the extra fat.
I've been known to wrap these up in small individual squares and
take them on trips with me. What could be better when a pang of
hunger strikes?*

2/3 cup semisweet chocolate chips

2 tablespoons unsalted butter

1 cup sugar

1 egg

1 egg white

1 (2½-ounce) container prune puree or ¼ cup pureed
dried plums

2 teaspoons vanilla extract

½ teaspoon salt

¾ cup all-purpose flour

⅓ cup unsweetened cocoa powder

Preheat the oven to 350°F. Line an 8-inch square baking
pan with aluminum foil, leaving an overhang at the sides.
Combine the chocolate and butter in the top of a double
boiler or a heat-safe bowl placed over a pan of simmering
water. Heat, stirring, until the mixture is smooth. Remove
the mixture from the heat and stir in the sugar, egg, egg
white, prune puree, vanilla, and salt, and stir until smooth.

Combine the flour and cocoa in a sieve, and sift into the
chocolate mixture. Stir just until blended, and pour into
the prepared pan. Bake until the top is firm to the touch

and a cake tester inserted in the center comes out with moist crumbs attached, about 30 minutes.

Cool the brownie slab completely in the pan on a wire rack. Using the overhang, lift the slab out of the pan and place on a cutting board. Slide it off the foil, and cut it into 16 squares.

MAKES 16 BROWNIES

TRAIL MIX

This great little snack takes 5 minutes to throw together, and it keeps a very long time if stored in a cool, dry place in an airtight container . . . perfect for travel, after a workout, anytime.

1 cup dried pineapple chunks

1 cup dried mango chunks

1 cup dried blueberries

1 cup dried cranberries

1 cup salted hulled sunflower seeds

1 cup semisweet chocolate chips or carob chips

1 cup shelled almonds

1 cup salted peanuts

1 cup coconut flakes

Combine all ingredients in a large bowl, and mix well.

MAKES 9 CUPS

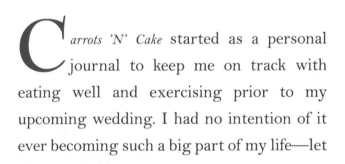

HAPPILY EVER AFTER?

C*arrots 'N' Cake* started as a personal journal to keep me on track with eating well and exercising prior to my upcoming wedding. I had no intention of it ever becoming such a big part of my life—let alone my job!

On the day that I quit my full-time job at Harvard, I made a pact with myself that I would succeed, and that quitting my cushy, well-paying job was a good decision. It's hard, but there are people who do it. Am I going to be poor? I seriously hope not, but you know what? I love what I do. I love every second of it. For the first time in a very, very long time I feel like I'm actually living.

The most frequent question I hear from friends, family, and the blogging community is this: How do you balance everything? I blog at *Carrots 'N' Cake*, work part-time at NuVal, write a weekly column for Health.com, plan an annual healthy-living summit for two hundred people, and do the social media and event promotion for a local wine and liquor company. Oh, yeah, and I wrote this book, too. How do I find the time to manage it all?

Honestly, you've gotta really want it . . . bad. I work insane hours. Most weeks, between my millions of jobs, I work close to sixty hours a week. When you have a blog where the content comes from the food you eat, you never stop working, and your brain never stops spinning with the thoughts of future blog posts. As a writer, you face rejection. Especially for someone like me, who is not naturally a writer, I face it all the time.

Being the Boss

Even though I technically consider blogging my job, it still feels like a hobby to me. I love it—probably because I am my own boss. While I do have a lot on my plate, I'm the one who decides what I do and when I do it. If I need a vacation day from answering comments or e-mails, I take it. If I want an extension on a blog project, I grant approval to myself. Sometimes I am overdue to get a blog post up, but I don't have the time or energy to post, so I make the executive decision to postpone it. Knowing that I am in control of this job takes a lot of the pressure off me.

It might seem that my life is work, work, work, all of the time, but I achieve balance by not writing about it all. There's a lot that happens between my breakfast and dinner posts that my readers don't see. I veg out and watch at least a couple of TV shows every night, but that rarely makes it into my blog commentary. Similarly, I take long walks with Mal and Murphy around the neighborhood, especially when the weather is nice, but when it comes to blog content, our walks aren't really interesting enough to put into a post. These pieces of my life are too mundane or personal to write about on my blog, but they are the fillers of time that separate online from real life. I could never do a reality show where I had cameras following me around all the time. That would drain everything from me. Blogging at least allows me to choose how much of my life is private, and while I do share most of it with my readers, there are some things that I just keep to myself.

Having Fun

I also think that I manage to balance it all because I try to keep it fun. I've gone through boring lulls on my blog, but the key is to find new motivation to keep creating interesting content. Nothing excites me more than coming up with a new recipe or fun event to share. Even a simple Question of the Day for my readers that stimulates conversation can transform the blog from me typing anonymously on a keyboard to a two-way intriguing discussion. The more interaction with readers I have, the more fun it is.

And of course, I have to stay organized to manage it all. Between my work as a full-time blogger, part-time NuVal employee, freelance writer, and social media guru, I stay superorganized with calendars, e-mail tags, and to-do lists.

Not only do I have everything color coded, but I delegate things to myself for the future in my online calendar. I even set up reminders to e-mail me when things are coming up so I can move them from the long-term list to the current list. I also rarely ever procrastinate!

I thought that my ultimate dream was to blog at *Carrots 'N' Cake* for a living. Basically, my blog would be my only source of income. But now that I've managed to juggle so much for so long, I wonder: Would I be happy with just one job?

GRATED CARROT CAKE

Carrots and *cake—the ultimate reward!*

---

2 cups all-purpose flour

2 cups granulated sugar

2 teaspoons baking powder

1 teaspoon baking soda

2 teaspoons ground cinnamon

1 teaspoon salt

1 cup canola or grapeseed oil

3 eggs, lightly beaten

2 teaspoons vanilla extract

3 cups shredded carrots (about 1¼ pounds)

1 cup chopped pecans

1 cup raisins

1 cup shredded unsweetened coconut

3/4 cup drained canned crushed pineapple

FOR THE FROSTING

1 (3-ounce) package cream cheese, softened

1 tablespoon butter, softened

1 teaspoon vanilla extract

2 cups sifted confectioners' sugar

Preheat the oven to 350°F. Grease a 13- by 9-inch baking pan with butter, line with parchment, and butter the parchment. Combine the flour, sugar, baking powder, baking soda, cinnamon, and salt in a sifter, mix well, and sift into

CONTINUED

a large bowl. Add the oil, eggs, and vanilla, and beat well. Fold in the carrots, pecans, raisins, coconut, and pineapple until mixed.

Scrape the batter into the prepared pan. Bake on a rack in the middle of the oven until the edges have pulled away from the sides of the pan and a cake tester inserted in the center comes out clean, about 1 hour. Cool the cake in the pan 10 minutes.

Meanwhile, make the frosting: Combine the cream cheese, butter, and vanilla in the bowl of an electric mixer and beat at low speed until fluffy. Beat in the confectioners' sugar at medium speed until fluffy.

Invert the cake onto a cake rack, remove the parchment, and cool completely. Place on a serving platter, and frost the top.

MAKES 12 SERVINGS

INDEX